The Joy of Half a Cookie

The Joy of Half a Cookie

Using Mindfulness to Lose Weight and End the Struggle with Food

Jean Kristeller, PhD,
with Alisa Bowman

A PERIGEE BOOK

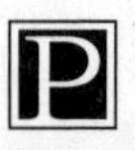

PERIGEE
An imprint of Penguin Random House LLC
375 Hudson Street, New York, New York 10014

ISBN: 978-0-399-17215-1

This book has been registered with the Library of Congress.

First edition: December 2015

PRINTED IN THE UNITED STATES OF AMERICA

3 5 7 9 10 8 6 4 2

Text design by Laura K. Corless

CONTENTS

Part One

The Science of Mindful Eating

Part Two

The Practice of Mindful Eating

PART ONE

The Science of Mindful Eating

CHAPTER ONE

An Introduction to Mindful Eating

Imagine what it would be like to lose weight *without* the struggle and *without* giving up your favorite foods, to be able to enjoy a glass of wine, a warm dinner roll, a slice of pizza, or a piece of chocolate *without* experiencing that familiar tug-of-war between your desire and your willpower. Think of how freeing it would be if you could truly savor a delicious treat without guilt and without worrying that, once you start, you won't be able to stop.

Is this possible? Could this become your reality? Yes, it can. Mindful eating will show you the way.

Before coming to my mindful eating workshops, the majority of women and men had lost anywhere from a few pounds to 50 pounds or more multiple times, depending on their body size and the type of diet they'd chosen. Depending on the plan, they had counted calories or points, feeling virtuous when they met their calorie goal—often 1,200 calories and sometimes as little as 500—and feeling awful when they missed, whether by only a little or by hundreds or even thousands of calories (though, by that time, they'd stopped counting). Some tolerated this good food–bad food approach for only a few days. But for others, it had worked well, at least for a while.

But then, inevitably, there came a point when they just couldn't stand to live like that anymore. Their old eating habits returned gradually, and so the pounds on the scale. Many couldn't even count the number of times this had happened to them. Often, they'd tell me that they just needed a little more self-control or willpower. One participant stands out clearly. On the first day, she told me, "I'm really good at 'no.' I say 'no' to so many things that, every once in a while, I want to consume all of it and never stop. And so that's what I do. Instead, I want to be good at 'yes.' I want to make friends with food."

She eventually learned to do just that, and now, in the pages of *The Joy of Half a Cookie*, it's my intention to show you how to do the same.

Say "Yes!" to Joy

Do you believe that forbidden foods—especially desserts, fried foods, snack chips, and cookies—contain an addictive combination of sweetness, fattiness, and/or saltiness, making them impossible to consume in small amounts? Assuming you're not too hungry, could you savor only half a cookie, a handful of corn chips, or a few spoonfuls of ice cream and put away the rest for another time? Could you put half a chocolate bar in your desk drawer—and then ignore it? Or would you be continually tempted to have just a little more?

As you read these words, you might be telling yourself, "That's impossible. No one can stop at just a few chips or a few bites of dessert." By the end of this book, after you've spent some time with the practices described in the second part of *The Joy of Half a Cookie*, it's my experience that you'll know it's possible because you'll have experienced this kind of freedom for yourself.

It doesn't matter how much out of control you might feel around certain foods at the moment. You can gain freedom. You really can.

That's because this is not like any other plan you've ever tried. In fact, when you embark on this plan, you are *not* going on a diet. Rather you are creating—and staying with—a new way of relating to food, to eating, to yourself, and to your body.

Based on the successful Mindfulness-Based Eating Awareness Training (MB-EAT) program I developed with funding from the National Institutes of Health (NIH) and have adapted into shorter workshops that I teach around the world, *The Joy of Half a Cookie* is about using mindfulness practice to give yourself permission to enjoy the foods you love, to choose the foods you enjoy, and to leave food on your plate if you don't want it or no longer feel like eating.[1] It's about self-care, self-nourishment, self-acceptance, kindness, exploration, and curiosity. It's about cultivating your inner gourmet rather than martialing your inner police force.

It has grown out of more than 30 years of experience and research in trying to help people learn to come into balance with their eating by linking their awareness with their desires. The underpinnings of this approach began decades ago with the understanding of how we can link our minds and bodies together, despite external pressures to do otherwise. It also draws on many years of research done both by myself and by a number of remarkable mentors and colleagues who've shared their wisdom and whose contributions I've attempted to honor in this book. Meditation practice, when made available to everyone, really can help us connect with the *inner wisdom* that leads us to handle complex choices, rather than trying to make them too simple, as many diets do.

Mindful eating is therefore about an entirely different way of looking at our relationship to our eating and food, one that pulls together a wide range of science-based perspectives on how our bodies and minds regulate themselves. It isn't about willpower or rigid self-control. Instead it's about creating balance through *self-care* and *self-regulation*. What's the difference? With willpower or self-control, you still want to keep on eating, but you force yourself to stop. With *self-regulation*, you check in mindfully, realize you're not hungry any more or aren't enjoying the food so much, so you simply decide to let it go. There's no struggle. You can always have more later, and you'll actually enjoy it more.

The core building blocks for the foundation of MB-EAT came together over a number of years, during my graduate studies and continuing beyond. The program now includes four core elements:

1. Meditation and mindfulness
2. The power of tuning in to your body and mind
3. Embracing, rather than fighting, the positive value of food
4. The power of science to show how these make a difference

Each of these elements melded together with my own personal experiences and struggle over many years. This chapter shares the story of how these building blocks came together slowly, gradually, to emerge into MB-EAT, and now, *The Joy of Half a Cookie*.

A Personal Struggle and a Scientific Journey

Throughout my teen and undergraduate years, I found myself in an endless round of self-deprivation during the day followed by over-eating almost every night, with strong feelings of guilt and shame fueling the cycle to start over again. Despite my attempts, I never lost the weight I'd hoped to—and in fact, I gained more. A familiar story.

After learning Transcendental Meditation and then studying abroad in Japan, I became interested in the newly emerging area of mind–body science. I then joined a cutting-edge research team at the University of Wisconsin that was exploring the effects of bio-feedback on people's ability to slow down their heart rate to help manage stress. I suggested meditation as another approach, and we found, to our surprise, that it was as effective or more so than bio-feedback in helping people slow their heart rates.[2] I became even more interested in how meditation might help link the mind and body, much as biofeedback does.

I was still struggling with my own eating and weight, avoiding carbohydrates, trying to apply the newly developing cognitive be-havioral therapy approaches both for myself and my clients, but not really succeeding, when I made another trip to Asia. There I became more aware of truly savoring my food (which was high in carbs), eating smaller portions, and to my surprise, effortlessly losing weight. I returned to the United States to continue graduate work at Yale University, where I promptly returned to my old eating habits and the weight came back on. At Yale I again began researching mind–body connections, also using biofeedback and meditation, but going beyond a simple relaxation model of meditation. Instead, the team was using an approach referred to as self-regulation, which cultivates the body's ability to heal itself rather than just focusing on taking away symptoms.[3] We asked the question, How could we help people reconnect the natural balance of the body and mind?

Just as exciting was the opportunity to work with researchers who were studying how people create their relationship to eating and food and how even "normal" eaters can lose touch with their experiences of physical hunger and fullness in the face of social pressures or other triggers to eat.[4] These researchers were also investigating the basic processes of taste experience and how this is affected by physical and psychological factors, such as hunger and being distracted.[5]

My thought was, Could I combine these two areas of science—self-regulation theory and perception of eating experience—to help individuals who were seriously struggling with their eating (and weight)? We couldn't apply electrodes to do biofeedback for hunger and satiety. But instead of telling my clients who were dealing with eating disorders to use a different diet, track everything they were eating, or just look for triggers to eating out of control, I began suggesting that they pay more attention to their physical hunger, relax their minds and bodies in the face of stress, choose to eat what they really liked, and stop eating when they'd had enough. I also began recommending that clients read Susie Orbach's groundbreaking book *Fat Is a Feminist Issue*, especially the chapter titled "The Experience of Hunger for the Compulsive Eater."[6]

I then began to wonder about trying this myself. If I gave myself permission to eat the foods that I loved earlier in the day, when I wasn't as hungry, would my taste buds perhaps tire and allow me to feel satisfied with just a reasonable amount? And what if I really paid attention to these experiences, if I slowed down and savored what I was eating, would the food also be more satisfying?

For one week, I gave myself permission to eat any sugary, fatty, high-calorie, sweet food I wanted for lunch. On the first day, I went straight to a nearby vending machine. I pressed the most tempting buttons. Down came the chips, and the chocolate cookies. They tasted pretty good, and I got through the rest of the day without thinking about food or hunger. I had my usual reasonable dinner and, much to my surprise, didn't want to eat anything more that evening.

On day two, I went back to the vending machine, made some different choices, and I still didn't want to raid the pantry after dinner. On day three, the vending machine didn't look appealing. I wanted something more indulgent. I walked to a bakery and got myself a large croissant and a piece of dark fudge chocolate cake. *Fantastic!* But I noticed something really important: The last few bites of the cake didn't taste quite as good as the first few, just as the research on taste was predicting.

On day four I was too busy to go to the bakery and nothing looked good in the vending machine. So I went around the corner to a pizza place, ordered two slices of my favorite, sat down, savored every bite, and again felt satisfied throughout the afternoon, but also a bit nervous. I hadn't had sweets at lunch. Would I feel an urge to empty the cookie shelf later that evening? To my surprise, I didn't.

By the end of the week, the message was clear. When I gave myself permission to eat my favorite, previously forbidden foods without guilt, I ate far less than I usually did at night, without any struggling. I found, to my amazement, I also enjoyed them more, but craved them less, and that I did not want to keep eating them endlessly. Soon these foods—the ones that I'd thought I'd never find the willpower or self-control to resist—lost much of their allure. It was a huge eye opener. I kept using this technique with patients, but it would be several years before I put the pieces of the puzzle together to create a mindfulness-based program.

Fast-forward a few years. Using meditation as part of therapy was becoming more acceptable and more popular. I had the opportunity to try out the pieces of the program I was developing in several more places, each of which added new insights. Using meditation with workers in a weight loss group at a factory in New Haven, Connecticut, gave me confidence that people with a wide range of backgrounds would be comfortable with a meditation-based program. Adapting the program for use at the Brown University Counseling and Psychological Services confirmed my own earlier experience with the power of mindful eating for letting go of weight concerns and struggles. And using it in the Department of Psychiatry at Cambridge Hospital, part of Harvard Medical School, made me less concerned that meditation might trigger psychiatric problems. The final pieces of the foundation dropped into place when I joined the faculty at the University of Massachusetts Medical Center in Worcester, which in the 1980s was at the forefront in the development of medical services incorporating mind–body components. In addition to other responsibilities, I began working with Jon Kabat-Zinn's ground-breaking Mindfulness-Based Stress Reduction (MBSR) program and helping with some of their research.[7] I was moving much closer to what has become MB-EAT today, offering a mindfulness-based program to individuals struggling with their eating and weight, finding that adding some of the MBSR components made it even more powerful.

But to do research with the program, I wanted to move back into a university psychology department. Shortly after beginning teaching at Indiana State University, one of our doctoral students, Brendan Hallett, asked to join the team, and we systematically began to assess the effects of the program for 18 women, ranging from 25 to 62 years, who were struggling with binge eating disorder and weight. None had ever meditated before. The results of this small study were very exciting and confirmed my clinical experience to that point: Frequency and size of binges dropped by more than half in a few weeks, and participants markedly decreased their overall struggle with eating; feelings of depression and anxiety also decreased. Further, the more these women used mindfulness practices with eating, the stronger the improvements they experienced.[8]

Encouraged by these positive results, my colleagues and I embarked on NIH-funded studies. The first one was a large study of men and women with binge eating disorder that included the capable involvement of Dr. Ruth Wolever at Duke University.[9] We were able to replicate the results from the first, smaller study. But we found it hard to predict who would be able to lose weight; while some people lost as much as 25 pounds in only a few months, others actually gained some weight, perhaps feeling that they were being given permission, for the first time, to eat whatever they wanted to. Again, the one clear predictor of success was how much they were actually using mindfulness practice.

So in our next NIH study, we decided to add on what has become a core part of the MB-EAT program: mindfully learning to tune in to calories, nutrition needs, and healthier food choices, which we refer to as cultivating *outer wisdom*. We also decided to design the program for individuals both with and without binge eating problems. The results were striking. By the end of the 10-week program, which this book is based on, study participants were dropping an average of 1 pound a week and maintaining that well after the program's end. Over time participants found it easier and easier to draw on "healthy restraint" in regard to food choices and with far less struggle.[10] In the last few years, we've found similar results in NIH-funded studies that have adapted the MB-EAT program to people with diabetes and those with less severe levels of weight issues.[11]

Participants vary in their weight loss. Some lose 20 or 25 pounds in the first few months. Others lose nothing at first, but then go on to drop more than 100 pounds after the formal program has ended.

Some don't lose very much, but their sense of struggle greatly diminishes. They no longer battle food or their urges to eat. By the end of the MB-EAT program, participants are able to balance their eating, eat mindfully, and experience true culinary joy and satisfaction. They are even able to do so when sitting inside a buffet-style restaurant with huge portions of highly tempting foods.

Here's more: Once participants learn how to become more mindful, some of the foods they once craved—the very foods they thought were too delicious to resist, that even seemed addicting—don't taste as nearly good or have lost their appeal entirely. So often a participant remarks, "I used to love these cookies/chips/donuts, but you know what? They're really not that good." It no longer takes willpower or self-control to stop eating these treats. They just don't want them anymore. They wait to indulge themselves with foods that are really worth eating!

On a personal note, this method has continued to help me completely let go of my own struggle. Using the techniques you're about to discover, I enjoy food more, eat less of it, and have ended the cycle of overeating, guilt, and deprivation. I hope you'll find success with it too.

It's Not About Willpower

When you attempt to lose weight by using willpower, you use external rules to guide your eating—only 1,200 calories a day, never take second helpings, and no desserts (except for fruit)—and then you try to force yourself to follow those rules. Think of a fresh baked cookie right from the oven, the one made from scratch using your grandmother's special recipe. Of course you want to eat it. Who wouldn't? I'll use the image of our hands to show the difference between willpower/self-control, and self-balance/self-regulation. As your hand reaches for that cookie, willpower is the other hand that wraps itself around your wrist and forcefully pulls it back. To strengthen your willpower, you might police yourself with food logs, diet buddies, weekly or daily weigh-ins, and negative self-talk, such as "No! I shouldn't."

When you attempt to lose weight with self-control, you manage your environment or change your thoughts so you don't have to exert so much willpower. To avoid feeling tempted by cookies or chips, you never buy them or, at the very least, never leave them out where you can see them. To prevent yourself from wanting larger servings, you opt for smaller bowls and plates or fool your body into feeling full by downing water before meals, eating lots of soup, or continually nibbling on so-called free foods you may not particularly enjoy. Maybe you avoid certain environments—buffets, restaurants that serve large portions, and potlucks. Think of that fresh baked cookie again. With self-control, your hands are clasped together at your lap. As long as they stay folded together like that, neither hand can reach for a cookie. This can be helpful and may even lead to new patterns—but may not help much when those cookies get left out on the counter, you're faced with a buffet, or everyone else is ordering dessert.

When you lose weight by cultivating balance and self-regulation, you can welcome that delicious cookie into your life. Self-regulation means you listen to the natural feedback systems within the body that send out the messages that your cells either need food or have had enough. You listen to the thoughts in your mind urging you on—and respond, rather than react, to them. You could choose to enjoy the cookie if you want it, when you're hungry or if it's a rare treat. Even if it's a huge cookie—the kind that might contain as many calories as an entire meal—there's no fear. You know that you'll be able to savor a few bites or perhaps half of it, wrapping up the other half for later when you'll be able to enjoy it all over again. There's a decision but no struggle. When you connect with your body and mind and engage your natural powers of self-regulation, your hands are open, welcome, and inviting, much as they are in the classic meditation posture. You can choose to take the cookie or you can leave it. You're using the wisdom of your body and your mind to make choices that are balanced, are easy, and surprisingly, require little effort.

It might be hard to imagine that you could ever manage your weight or your eating in this way, but you really can, and mindfulness will show you how.

How Mindfulness Helps You Lose Weight

Mindfulness meditation is *not* just about relaxing, although that can happen. It is about tuning in, letting go of judgment, and embracing what you experience in the moment. Practicing meditation helps cultivate our capacity to stay mindful, regardless of how compelling or overwhelming a situation feels, and will help you to lose weight and keep it off in two key ways.

Tuning in to your inner wisdom. By becoming more mindful, you'll tap into an *inner wisdom* that helps you sense how physically hungry you are, how full you feel, and when a food's flavor is disappearing and is no longer enjoyable enough to keep on eating. Inner wisdom includes learning to recognize and honor how to use food for comfort, relaxation, and celebration, without going overboard. Rather than forcing yourself not to take second helpings, you'll let your wisdom be your guide. You ask yourself questions like "Do I really want this? Would I really enjoy it? Am I really hungry? Am I still enjoying this?" Your answers help you decide whether you want that next bite or an additional helping. As a result you'll find that three or four bites might be just as satisfying—and will leave you much less uncomfortable—as one or two servings.

Tuning in to your outer wisdom. Rather than adopting someone else's rules about calories or nutrition, you'll use *outer wisdom* to inform your own choices. There's so much information about nutrition and exercise out there that it can feel overwhelming. One day you learn that fatty foods are fattening. The next you hear certain types of fat are actually slimming, but other fats are not. One day you read that you should be a vegetarian or vegan for optimal health. The next you're told that carbs should be avoided.

With *The Joy of Half a Cookie*, you'll be encouraged to explore this nutritional information, consulting your physician or a dietician if you have particular health needs. Then you'll use this input to inform your own wisdom about the types of foods and the amounts of foods your body really needs, for weight loss, weight management, and overall health. On this plan, you don't split foods into two categories: foods I'm allowed to eat and foods I'm not allowed to eat. Rather, there are simply foods you enjoy more and foods you enjoy less, and foods that are healthier for you and foods that are less nutritious, especially in larger quantities. Food as "medicine," perhaps; food as "poison," no.

But calories (which I refer to as *food energy*) do count, and learning what is a good balance for you is a path to freedom. You'll discover how to become attentive and relaxed, rather than obsessive and anxious, about how you're balancing your eating and your body's need for fuel (food energy). And you'll gradually shift away from your current eating patterns—the ones that you've had for years and that keep coming back after every diet—to new patterns that can work for you long term.

By employing both types of wisdom—inner and outer—you'll bring your eating and your life into balance.

As you do so, you'll be able to do the following:

Let go of the struggle. People tell me that, before learning to eat mindfully, it seemed to them as if they spent most of their waking moments worrying about food and their weight: what to eat, what not to eat, when to eat, how much to eat, and what effect it would have on the scale. With mindfulness, you'll learn to let go of this seemingly constant struggle and give this energy and attention to areas of your life that are richer and more important than whether you're going to eat that brownie.

The patterns you have and the way you relate to food have been there a long time. It might take some time to re-create them, but you can begin to experience success immediately, which then continues over time, as it did for Mary. I ran into her about a year after she'd attended one of my workshops. She began to tell me how excited she was about being able to have ice cream back in the house. She used to binge on whole quarts of it, and for a few months after the workshop, she wouldn't have any in the house, just treating herself occasionally to some at restaurants or to an ice cream cone—really savoring it and enjoying it. Then she'd found she could have one of her less favorite flavors in the house (vanilla or strawberry). But recently, she had discovered she could have her favorite (mint chocolate chip) and eat it only a few spoonfuls at a time.

Turn mindless eating into mindful eating. Our decisions around eating can happen in milliseconds: I want more. I want less. I'm terrible for doing this so I'm going to keep doing it. If I have this I'll feel better about myself. Even as we're obsessing, we're often not even aware we are making decisions. By becoming aware, we can interrupt the cycle and gain freedom over the next moment. We can change our automatic reactions into mindful response. Through meditation practice and mindful observation, you'll learn how to notice what's arising in a nonjudgmental way. You'll get in touch with what it means to be hungry, full, satisfied, and filled with pleasure, rather than with discomfort. You'll learn how to make decisions around your eating that are enriching rather than painful. We are bombarded with a wealth of choices. You'll learn how to stop and tune in to that wealth of choices without being overwhelmed and without drawing unnecessary boundaries.

Notice the thoughts that trip you up. We bring a history to every meal we eat. For example, workshop participants tell me that they struggle to leave food on their plates because their mothers always told them not to waste food. When I ask, "Is your mother in the room?" some even joke, "Oh, she's here all right." I then ask, "I wonder if there are other things your mother told you to do, that you don't do anymore?" And suddenly the room is quiet for a moment. Then I hear a chorus of, "Oh yes."

With this book, you'll learn how to feel comfortable leaving food on your plate no matter what your real or imagined mother tells you. And you'll notice and respond to other unhelpful thoughts that powerfully affect your eating. How many times have you lost the battle between your willpower and your desire and told yourself, "I'll just have a little bit"? Then maybe you had a little bit more. Then you thought, "I've blown it," and you kept eating until you felt physically uncomfortable or even sick? The "I've Blown It" cycle often reflects a sense of defeat: I can't control myself anyway, so why bother? The secret to overcoming the cycle has nothing to do with shoring up your willpower. Reactions get locked in and you might feel as if you didn't have a choice, but with the power of mindfulness, you do. When you give yourself permission to be present with strong negative emotions, cravings, guilt, and other triggers as well as to enjoy the foods you love, you can gradually break this cycle, tap into your inner wisdom, and feel a sense of freedom when you eat.

Get away from the food police. The idea of policing yourself—whether with a journal, a buddy, or the scale—often triggers a sense of rebellion and an inner voice that whispers, "Who says I can't have this?" With mindfulness, you'll shift away from policing yourself and toward understanding and nurturing yourself. Can it be helpful to keep track of your food sometimes? Yes, and I'll show you in Chapter 6 how to do it in a totally different way, with a sense of curiosity and exploration, rather than as if someone were looking over your shoulder.

Let go of calorie anxiety. I've worked with some people who fear calories so much that they don't even like saying the word and never check to see how much they're eating. Others obsess over minor amounts like 10 or 20 calories, counting up what they've eaten every day. With *The Joy of Half a Cookie*, you'll learn to manage your eating more flexibly, in much the same way as you manage your money if you're on a budget—not an absolute set amount every day, but keeping an eye on the bottom line.

My Wish for You

There's a cartoon I like to share during my workshops. It's of Cathy, the guilt-ridden comic strip character, created by Cathy Guisewite, who struggles with food, love, family, and work. She's tied herself to a chair to help resist the power of a box of cookies on the floor nearby, but she's still reaching out for those cookies with one foot. Whenever I show this cartoon, everyone laughs. That's because this is almost a universal struggle. You are not alone in this struggle, and you can free yourself from it.

After researching the psychology of eating, studying mindfulness meditation, and teaching these skills to hundreds of clients and workshop participants over more than two decades, there's something I now know with deep conviction: Everyone can improve his or her relationship to eating and food, enjoy delicious foods more, and find the way to a smaller body size, with less and less struggle over time.

You really can enjoy just half a cookie for dessert or a few chips for a snack. You can navigate big holiday dinners without anxiety, and you can put the word *comfort* back in "comfort food." You can also go to a party where dozens of foods are being presented, and you can feel a sense of freedom that comes from knowing that you're not going to overdo it. You can eat smaller portions and paradoxically create more satisfaction.

You may not be able to do all of this today and you may not be able to do it by next week or next month, but you can learn and practice important skills that will eventually make the kinds of experiences that I just described your norm rather than the exception. You can drop pounds, and keep them off, without feeling deprived and without missing out on everything you love about eating.

Rather than having a relationship with pain and anxiety, you can cultivate a relationship with flavor, nourishment, and satisfaction. You'll reconnect to savoring and enjoying, to letting go of the struggle, and to welcoming the taste and the pleasure of eating. It's possible. *The Joy of Half a Cookie* will show you how.

Let's get started.

CHAPTER TWO

Cultivating the Habit of Mindful Eating

The Joy of Half a Cookie is based on several decades of research—completed by myself and others—that has explored the psychological influences on overeating. It includes a blend of many different approaches, yet mindfulness serves as the foundation for the entire plan.

Mindfulness may be a new catch phrase, but it points toward a universal truth: Much of our struggle and suffering in life comes from over-attachment to things we think we want, linked with fear of things that might cause problems. Mindfulness allows us to release some of that struggle by simply observing this reactive self and considering other possibilities.

And mindfulness is for everyone. Though it draws from ancient Buddhist practices, it's something we can *all* do—regardless of our spiritual beliefs—if we just stop, pay attention, and cultivate awareness and appreciation of the moment rather than just reacting. The mindfulness seed is within you. It is a basic human capacity. All you need is the intention to cultivate it. Mindfulness isn't something that requires many years of study. You don't need to believe in reincarnation or karma. Nor must you have a yoga mat or sit cross-legged on the floor to do it. I've taught mindfulness to people of all backgrounds and religions. No matter your current issues with food or weight and no matter your religious beliefs, mindfulness practice can help you transform your relationship with food and your body.

Try This Now

You may worry that you don't have what it takes to be mindful. Let me reassure you. You've been mindful before, many times throughout your life. Now think back over your day, your week, or your month. Have you stopped and appreciated a sunset or beautiful rainbow? Or looked into the face of a baby? Or stopped to smell a flower? If not, then find one this week. You don't have to put words to the experience or judge it or worry about how you are going to respond. You are just there. When this happens, that's mindfulness.

What Is Mindfulness?

When you practice mindfulness, you don't try to become mindful of every single experience, but you do focus on the ones that matter the most. You deliberately pay attention, without judgment, both to your *inner world*—your bodily sensations (such as hunger and taste, among many others), your emotions, your thoughts—and to your *outer world* (for instance, the nutrition value of that favorite snack food in front of you).

Mindfulness can be cultivated in the moment, but only when you choose to bring your attention to something you value. Once you do so, you may be surprised at how much richer the experience is. Consider any routine task, ranging from driving your car to walking down the street to gardening. What happens when your mind wanders? Do your thoughts immediately fly off to negative self-judgment? To fantasies? To other tasks? Do you enjoy the experience at hand? Do you do it well? Or do you get lost, pull up something that wasn't a weed or start the dishwasher but forget to put the soap in?

Now consider what happens when you bring your mindful awareness to a task. You probably already do this occasionally. Maybe you become totally absorbed as you enjoy the sounds of crickets, the color of new buds on a plant, or something more complex, such as being absorbed in a shopping trip for something you really need. This is what mindfulness can be like.

But as with any skill, mindfulness improves with cultivation, and that's where meditation practice makes a difference. By sitting in meditation, you'll strengthen your ability to remain mindful—during conversations, while driving, and, especially, while eating. Sitting and following your breath in and out with your mind sharpens your ability to pay attention, tune in, and be aware. The skill of tuning in to the breath teaches you how to tune in to your hunger, your fullness, your emotions, your cravings, your enjoyment, and more. The skill of mindfulness is placing your attention where you wish it to go—not necessarily where it's pulled to in the moment.

Mindfulness also teaches you to go even deeper and get in touch with what I call the *wise mind*. Think of the mind as having levels of quality of thought. On the surface is the *wandering* or *chattering mind*: those thoughts about plans for the day, shopping lists, or almost random thoughts and memories that seem to swirl around, much like overhearing bits of conversation at a party. The wandering mind, which has become the focus of considerable research, can pull us into worries and concerns, but also into the deeper *thinking mind*, assessing, reflecting, problem solving, perhaps pondering some issue in our life.[1] When these types of thoughts quiet down, we can engage with the wise mind, when new perspectives appear to arise that feel more integrative, creative, compelling, or somehow more grounded or truthful. Exciting new neuroscience evidence is showing that with experience, meditators have increasing control over the wandering mind, and greater access to the integrative functioning in the frontal parts of their brains, a sign that meditation, even for beginners, can have power to create distinct experiences of peace, calmness, wisdom, and insight.[2] This can happen in every domain of our being: our thought processes, our emotions, our decisions, our relationships, our spiritual life.[3]

Drawing on the wise mind is especially important when it comes to eating. Normally much of our eating seems automatic. Yet those decisions can also involve all aspects of who we are. While we certainly make thoughtful choices—for example, what foods to cook or order off a menu or choose out of the refrigerator or cupboard—we are often barely aware of the considerations that go into making these choices. And yet individuals with relatively little meditation experience may have powerful insights on how to handle a difficult food choice, when they let go of their usual chattering or wandering minds for even a few moments.

Breaking the Habit of Mindless Eating

Mindfulness is a habit, one that *The Joy of Half a Cookie* will help you to develop. Practicing mindful eating will help you weaken the more common pattern of mindless eating.

Think of what happens when you order a tub of popcorn at the movies. You bring it to your seat. You sit down. Then your hand continually travels from the tub to your mouth and back again, mostly without your awareness. Because you're absorbed by the movie, you probably don't take much time to notice how the popcorn tastes. You just eat.

And then, eventually, your hand reaches the bottom of the tub, roots around for some kernels, and finds none. This can even happen when the popcorn is old and stale, as Brian Wansink, head of the Cornell University Food and Brand Lab, has shown in one of his studies.[4] Depending on the size of the popcorn bucket, you may have just eaten 1,200 calories, the equivalent of two personal pan pepperoni pizzas. Yet you're left with a sense of longing, as if you didn't get enough.

If we ate mindlessly only at the movies, it might not be such a problem, but we tend to eat mindlessly much of the time. We walk by a coworker's candy jar and we grab a piece of chocolate. We're sitting next to a loved one who happens to be eating chips. We grab a few, and then more, even though we're not hungry. We finish the rather large serving of lasagna because it's there.

We're surrounded by many influences to eat, and our reactions are triggered rapidly. Just the sight, smell, or thought of food can lead us to the cookies, chips, or snack bowl, allowing us to insert hundreds and even thousands of excess calories into our mouths but not truly enjoy most of them. Or we're flung into struggle as part of us is pulled forward and the other part resists.

Worse, mindless eating often leaves us feeling unsatisfied, even emotionally empty, and yet at the same time uncomfortably full. That's because, when we eat mindlessly, we remain out of touch with the signals our bodies give us. Our bodies communicate with us all the time, giving us important input that we can respond to with wisdom as long as we learn to listen. If we don't pay attention, though, we remain out of touch with our hunger, our fullness, and, as important, our enjoyment.

Mindless eating also keeps us in the dark about nutritional value. Do you know roughly how many calories (food energy) were in your lunch? Was it what you needed to get through the afternoon to dinner? Or far less, if you had a light salad? Or perhaps far more, if you went to a fast-food place and super-sized it? Do you know how much your body needs to maintain your weight? To lose a pound? To gain one? How many calories would your body need to stay at the weight you hope to get to?

When we react without considering what we are doing, we also end up feeling a loss of control and a loss of choice. This leads to anxiety, depression, eating disorders, and addictive behavior. That's partially because mindless eating often includes mindless thinking. When we encounter a trigger to eat—whether it's visual, mental, or social—we react with a thought (or several thoughts), many of which take place so quickly that we're unaware of them. An endless array of thoughts are capable of triggering a destructive cycle of overeating, whether a relatively small amount or a true binge. We often don't even realize what we are telling ourselves, such as "One bite won't hurt." Some of these thoughts are understandable. Others are just habits that we use to justify the first bite, the next bite, and then many more.

One of the worst aspects of mindless eating is that as it causes you to eat more, it also lessens your enjoyment. This might have worked when we lived in a culture with few choices, without abundant food, with most people having the need to simply fuel their bodies to get through hours of heavy manual labor, but that's not the world most of us live in today.

Breaking the Habit of Restricted Eating

Perhaps you're reading this, saying to yourself, "I wish I could be mindless. Instead I think about every bite I eat, every meal, every day." That's restricted eating, the dieting mind-set that makes you hyperaware of every morsel you put in your mouth and that causes you to sort foods into the black and white categories of "Yes, I can eat that" vs. "No, I can never have that."

No sugar
No fried foods
No butter
No meat
No dairy
No packaged or processed foods
No gluten

Likely you've heard or read that these foods contain an addictive combination of salt, fat, and sugar, or that they lead to heart disease, diabetes, and other health problems. Similarly, you may have read or experienced that certain environments—such as buffets and all-you-can-eat restaurants—encourage overeating, and that we should all just stay away from such places.

Maybe you've decided to forgo certain foods or environments after careful reflection and for good personal reasons, and there is no struggle involved. You might even find these kinds of rules make your life easier. We're bombarded with food-related choices: Should I have bacon and eggs or oatmeal? A burger or a salad? Pasta or broccoli? Strict diets can simplify this kind of decision-making because then many foods fall into the "no" category. And abstinence can indeed decrease the pull of particular foods, but only if approached with an attitude of truly letting go, rather than trying to hold on.

For many, however, the "no" mind-set can be extremely limiting. We live in a world packed full of tempting foods and eating environments. They are difficult to avoid. Perhaps you are able to avoid buffet-style restaurants, but what are you going to do during the next potluck book club event? If you take a cruise? Or go on a yoga retreat, where the food, even though nutritious, is served buffet-style? Will you also avoid networking events where a wide variety of foods are served? For most of us, it's not realistic to eat only at home, to keep all tempting foods out of the house, and to never go near restaurants that pump the smell of fried food into the air.

This restricted eating mind-set reduces the enjoyment of eating, socializing, and to some degree, life. Because of all the "no" foods on their lists, many restricted eaters find it challenging to eat with friends or allow someone else to cook them a meal. I once chatted with a woman who told me she had always wanted to travel to Japan but had just heard that most Japanese meals include white rice. Because she had decided never to eat white rice again, she was disappointed that she could never go to that country. She had made an entire region of the world off limits due to her own inflexible eating habits.

A New Earth author Eckhart Tolle wrote, "Whatever you fight, you strengthen, and what you resist, persists."[5] Perhaps you've experienced this for yourself. As soon as you tell yourself, "No more sugar ever," what happens? You start thinking about foods that contain sugar! The more you resist, the stronger your desire. Eventually your desire overwhelms your ability to resist. You go off a diet and quickly shift from hyperawareness to the opposite end of the spectrum: mindlessness. You stop choosing carefully and stop counting calories and the weight comes back on.

This sorting of foods into "okay to eat" and "not okay to eat" causes us unnecessary pain and struggle. Restricted eaters are often mired in self-judgment: positive when keeping to their restrictions and negative when they don't ("I'm bad for eating this." "I shouldn't have that." "I'm weak if I let myself have this."). And the restrictive "no" mind-set also gives the food all the power. Patterns in our brains are driven by awareness and attention and are strengthened by desire and aversion. So once that strong desire is there, we can't get rid of it by continually struggling with it. With truly physiologically addictive substances—such as nicotine, alcohol, or most drugs—abstinence may be the only answer. But my experience with so-called food addiction is that it is almost entirely psychological in nature.[6] Do pleasurable foods affect our brain, increase dopamine, lead to craving? Unquestionably. But these foods do this for just about everyone, whether they have a sense of being addicted or not.

There is a middle way between mindless eating and restricted eating. It's not about shifting back and forth between one and the other. It's about finding the balance between these two extremes, where flexibility, conscious choice, and enjoyment meet. When you identify the foods you crave the most and learn to savor those foods mindfully, something amazing and powerful happens: You are able to enjoy those foods for the first time. Rather than eat three sugar doughnuts in a rush—without truly tasting a single bite and while feeling guilty and remorseful the whole time—you'll be able to eat just half a doughnut while savoring every single bite of the experience. Mindfulness brings attention and awareness while interrupting the pull or push of those highly conditioned reactions, so the natural self-regulation processes of the body can play the role they are designed to do.

And all of this allows you to have experiences like Bob told me about. He and a friend often visited all-you-can-eat buffets. Some people have drinking buddies. Bob had an eating buddy. He and his friend overate together, and they looked forward to it. But he'd become concerned about his weight, which is why he came to our program.

Many diet experts would have cautioned Bob, telling him to give up buffets altogether because they were too dangerous, filled with temptations that no dieter could ever resist.

Instead I helped him find a way to enjoy his favorite pastime and still lose weight. By the end of the program, Bob was still going to buffets, and he was still hanging out with his friend. But now he was losing weight. What changed? Bob was no longer overeating when he went to these restaurants. He was merely sampling and savoring smaller amounts of the foods that called to him the most, and he was loving every single bite of them.

Cultivating the Habit of Mindful Eating

Mindful eating is the middle way between mindless eating and restricted eating, and it's based on several principles.

PRINCIPLE 1

Only *You* Know What Your Mind and Body Needs

No one can tell you how hungry you feel or when you've eaten enough to feel full. Your friends don't know how much you need to eat to feel satisfied. Neither does the chef in the restaurant kitchen. Nor does any popular diet.

Once you tap into your inner wisdom—informed by your hunger, satisfaction, and enjoyment—and balance it with outer wisdom—informed by knowledge about food energy and nutrition—you'll make the wise, but flexible decisions for your health, your weight, and your life.

PRINCIPLE 2

You'll Use Your Thoughts and Feelings to Inform Yourself, Not Punish Yourself

Rather than constantly being caught up in "shoulds" and "shouldn'ts," you'll learn from the practices in Part Two of this book to open yourself up to the way your body, your eating habits, your desire for certain foods, your cravings, and your moods really are, rather than the way you think they *should* be. Rather than reacting to such things, you'll simply notice them with nonjudgmental awareness. This awareness will help you make wiser decisions about whether you really want a food and how much of it will satisfy you.

PRINCIPLE 3

There Are No Bad Foods

Yes, some foods might contain more nutrients than others, but no foods are completely off limits (unless they need to be, for you). When part of a balanced diet, small tastes of your favorite foods do not lead to weight gain or disease. You really can indulge (modestly), without guilt. There are no absolutely right or wrong foods to eat, but rather varying degrees of value and satisfaction from what you choose.

PRINCIPLE 4

Calories Do Count

While inner wisdom will go a long way to helping you feel satisfied with fewer calories, your success hinges on developing outer wisdom, too. If you are on a budget, you probably don't track every single purchase, but you do look at price tags, comparison shop, and have a general idea of whether you can afford something. You'll soon learn how to do the same with eating. If you know about the energy value in the foods you eat or want to eat, your own energy needs, and the health effects of certain foods, you'll be able to make wiser decisions about which foods and how much are most appropriate for you and why. You'll be able to choose foods you love in amounts that satisfy, while you opt to forgo other foods that you don't love or need quite as much.

PRINCIPLE 5

Your Inner and Outer Wisdoms Work Together

These two wisdoms blend together, and arise from being mindful so you'll be able to focus your mind in productive ways. By being gently aware of your thoughts, emotions, and triggers to eat as they arise, you'll create space to consider what you wish to do about them. Sometimes you may decide to eat a little bit. Sometimes you might decide to eat more. The choice will vary from moment to moment and situation to situation, with mindfulness as your guide.

PRINCIPLE 6

Relying on Willpower and Guilt Leads to Dissatisfaction and Struggle

Exchange willpower and guilt for exploration and understanding, and invite yourself to get in touch with all of the thoughts and emotions—positive and negative—that call up a desire to eat.

PRINCIPLE 7

You'll Always Have a Relationship with Food

Whether it's a positive one or a negative one depends on the state of mind you bring to every bite.

PRINCIPLE 8

Joy Can Be Found in Every Bite

When you become mindful, you can bring joy back into every bite, as you savor your experience, nurturing yourself and respecting the food that brings you life and energy.

PRINCIPLE 9

Your Life Is About Much More Than How You Eat

It's my hope that, with the practices in this book, you'll develop a relationship with food that is nourishing and in balance with the rest of your life. Rather than being in a constant struggle, you'll experience a sense of freedom, knowing that you are the one who is in charge and recognizing that your life is about far more than your concerns about eating or your weight. And that those other areas of your life may deserve more of your awareness, attention, and appreciation.

Mindful Eating Is . . .

Deliberately paying attention to your experience of food and eating, without judgment.

Becoming aware in each moment, both internally (your thoughts, emotions, hunger, flavor, fullness) and externally (nutritional value of various foods).

Appreciating the difference between physical hunger and other triggers for eating, such as strong emotions, thoughts, and social pressures.

Choosing to eat foods as much as possible that you enjoy *and* that nourish your body.

Experiencing the flavor of a food as it shifts and evolves from one bite to the next.

Noticing how fullness develops in your stomach and how you feel once you've eaten enough.

Using information about the nutritional value and energy of food to meet your personal needs and inform your choices of what and how much to eat.

Freeing energy from worries about food and giving it to other important areas of your life.

CHAPTER THREE

Connecting with True Hunger

What Leads You to the First Bite

Have you ever found yourself standing in the kitchen, your hand buried in a bag of chips, your mouth full of salty crunchiness, and then wondered, "How did I get here?" Or maybe, during a reception, someone walked by with a tray filled with fried morsels. You grabbed one and put it in your mouth. Then another came by. And another. You were not necessarily grabbing them because of true hunger. Nor because they looked delicious and you wanted them. You were eating them simply because they were there.

Some of your eating might be so automatic that you don't even remember doing it. Chances are, if I asked you to think back over your day and tell me what you've eaten, you wouldn't be able to remember all of it. Perhaps you'd recall your main meals, but how about the piece of chocolate your coworker offered to you just before a meeting? It's likely that you regularly consume a couple hundred calories every day, if not more, that you just don't remember.

That's how mindless our eating really can be.

We make on average 200 to 300 food-related decisions a day and, most often, we're aware of how we make those decisions for only a small percentage of them, according to my colleague Brian Wansink at Cornell University.[1] Wansink has spent much of his career conducting fascinating studies about the triggers that lead to mindless eating. Everything from the size of our dinner plates to the social context to our moods and thoughts can affect when we eat, what we eat, and how much we eat—often without our mindful awareness.

The triggers might be visual, such as those homemade brownies that a coworker left in the break room or that free sample offered at the store. Or maybe they awake your other senses: the scent of your neighbor's grilled steak or those crunching sounds coming from your office mate's cubicle. They come in the form of social pressure, when everyone else at your table orders an appetizer or your friend hands you a glass of wine. They often arise out of habit, such as that ice cream you eat every evening or the dinner you eat every day at about the same time, whether you are hungry or not. And eating can be self-soothing in nature—such as when you reach for food to satisfy a desire for comfort.

These eating triggers are endless, which is why getting rid of them or avoiding them commonly backfires. Sure, you can keep overly tempting foods out of the house. Or you can carefully wrap up and store away the cookies and chips. But you can't eliminate triggers everywhere you go. No matter how careful you are, you will encounter situations where food has been left out. It will be offered to you at parties, and its aroma will waft toward you as you shop or head to your seat at the movies.

Alternatively, you can learn to listen to the cues your body provides when your cells need energy, primarily eating when you're physically hungry—which may still be at the party, in the mall, or at the movies. Connecting with true physical hunger is one of the most powerful brakes for mindless eating.

What Is Physical Hunger?

Hunger is natural and normal. Think of it as a helpful signal that your body has been using stored energy.

When blood sugar drops, physical hunger rises. Initially, it might feel like a mildly empty feeling or gnawing in your abdomen. If no new food energy comes in, the body shifts to burning stored energy for fuel, dampening hunger for a while. Eventually, though, the signals will come back stronger than before. At this point, the hunger might feel urgent and intense. In addition to that gnawing in your stomach, you might also be light-headed or jittery.

These sensations are just your body's way of telling you that your gastrointestinal (GI) tract has finished processing your last meal and that cells throughout your body need more glucose to burn for energy. Every cell in your body needs food energy every day. Failing to tune in to these signals can happen for various reasons. It may be that you've just never really noticed them, or you've been on many strict diets that have disconnected you even more from them, or perhaps you're in the middle of a high-stress period that demands your attention over everything else.

When we eat mindlessly, it's hard for us to tell the difference between physical hunger and other sensations that can feel a lot like the real thing. Thirst, for some people, can feel like hunger. Our bodies also become conditioned to feeling hungry regardless of whether we truly need more calories. So if you've had a snack at 11 a.m., you may still experience your stomach growling at noon if that's when you usually have lunch (and this is when outer wisdom can be helpful, as you realize you might want to delay lunch for a while that day).[2]

I've found that some people reach for food so quickly that they never register even those initial rumblings. I ask them, "What does physical hunger feel like to you?" They tell me that they just don't know. Instead, they graze all day, continually feed their cells more and more fuel. Others tell me that they are afraid of becoming too hungry, eating large amounts as soon as they feel even a slight twinge of hunger. Others, usually chronic dieters, have tuned out hunger. Regardless of your pattern, becoming fully mindful of physical hunger may take some time, but most people, I've found, can begin to do so fairly quickly.

Other Reasons We Eat

Simply put, the desire for food can be confused with physical hunger and can arise for all types of reasons, including the following:

Seeing food. The sight and smells of delicious food can make us feel hungry, even when we've just eaten. This is similar to Pavlov's dog learning to salivate at the sound of a bell. Our mouths salivate when we see cookies, cake, and other treats, even when we've just had a big meal. Even just thinking about food, listening to someone tell you about a delicious food, or seeing television commercials that depict food may be enough to rev up your desire to eat.

Memories. Part of why you love chocolate chip cookies may date back to experiences of eating your mother's home-baked ones. So even a poor-quality processed chocolate chip cookie has some appeal as you pursue the traces of experience buried deep in your mind. Or the memories may be more complex. I once counseled a woman who often stopped at a particular fast-food restaurant and always ordered fries. She wanted to cut down on them, so she went from super-sizing them to the small order, but was resisting leaving them off her order entirely. This seemed puzzling because, by this point, she admitted she really didn't like them so much, yet found herself strongly pulled toward them. After we talked about it, she realized that the fries were serving as a reminder of her daughter, who had died in an accident a few years before and who had loved to eat them. With this realization, she was first able to eat just a few, leaving the rest, and then was able to let go of ordering the fries as often.

Social pressure. Sometimes we eat because everyone else is. Maybe you're out with friends. You're not hungry, but then someone wants to stop for ice cream. You think, "I don't want to be the only person left out," so you order a cone, too. Or maybe you're at your mother-in-law's home and she brings out homemade brownies and presses you to eat several. And you eat them, reluctantly, because you think refusing would hurt her feelings. Once you cultivate more mindfulness, you might say, after the first one, "Your brownies are always so delicious, but I'm really full. Could I bring one home with me?"

Talking ourselves into eating. We sometimes justify eating with thoughts that we're barely aware of, for example, "I'll just have a bite." Have you ever said that to yourself? If so, were you really planning on having only one bite? Or does it really mean, "I'm going to eat as much as I want"? Similarly, the thought, "Just a little bit won't hurt," could be true if you have this thought only once a week or so. But when you tell yourself this multiple times a day, that thought can add up to thousands of extra calories over the week.

Another common thought, especially for chronic dieters, is, "I feel like being bad." This one harkens all the way back to our upbringing. In the early 1960s, psychiatrist Eric Berne wrote the bestseller *Games People Play*, which brilliantly describes three competing ego states: child, adult, and parent.[3] The inner parent is the caregiver but also the rule maker. The inner adult is wise, emotionally balanced, and flexible. And the inner child is willful, fun loving, and spontaneous. Berne makes the point that we have all three of these elements inside of us, and they can cause inner conflict. Your inner child might sneak a cookie with the thought, "I feel like being bad" or "You can't tell me what to do" or even "No one has to know." Then, as you are eating, your inner parent scolds your inner child with critical thoughts, "What's wrong with you?" and "Why don't you have any self-control?" Sound familiar?

The solution *isn't* to ignore such thoughts. Nor is it to battle them. Rather, it's to become mindfully aware of them. As you work with mindful eating, you may find that "I'll just have a bite" shifts from opening a dangerous door to opening a window to being mindful about the experience of that one bite. The amazing thing about food is that we can have only one bite and then decide, mindfully, that that is indeed all we want or need. Similarly, "I feel like being bad and rebellious" can serve as a signal to consider, "What could my inner child and inner adult agree on right now?" Perhaps the playful inner child and the flexible inner adult will instead embrace the cookie, enjoy it—and show the inner parent that they don't need five more.

The Hunger for Comfort

Many people reach for high-calorie foods as a form of comfort during times of stress, sadness, anger, anxiety, boredom, fatigue, and depression—the list goes on. Sometimes the emotion is apparent, but often it can take some mindfulness to recognize it.

Consider Clare, one of my clients. She had recently retired and had been taking care of her grandchildren during the day, keeping herself very busy. But then Clare's daughter had been laid off and was keeping her children home with her. Clare's days now suddenly felt empty, and she was finding herself much more frequently fixing herself snacks during the day out of boredom.

Upon further reflection, she realized that it also involved anxiety and depression about some other issues in her life that she'd been distracted from by taking care of the children. Clare made a list of other activities to consider whenever she experienced such feelings, especially if she found herself in the kitchen. She then began reminding herself, "Oh right, I'm not hungry . . . instead, I can work on my photography, my scrapbooking, or just surf the net." Although the other issues also needed attention, she was able to keep from regaining the weight that had gradually been coming off.

Another client, Karen, found that she often ate during the afternoon at work. "I really am hungry," she told me. With mindfulness, though, she realized that in reality, she was usually confusing anxiety related to work demands with hunger and that her eating was a way of procrastinating. Eating put off difficult work tasks as well as her anxiety about them. With this new understanding, she began to take a short self-care break whenever she felt the urge to procrastinate. Rather than eating, she went to a list of alternatives, including reading something relaxing or just walking around the office area, allowing ideas to percolate. She also found that she could *surf the urge* to eat, a concept developed by Alan Marlatt to help individuals with serious alcohol problems use mindfulness to resist cravings for a drink.[4] She discovered she could sit mindfully with the sensation of stress or desire for a snack, and that, much like a wave in the ocean, the feelings peaked and then ebbed, eventually disappearing. If she just rides it out, she now knows that the uncomfortable feeling goes away, no eating required.

Even though we're reaching for comfort from food, many of us almost immediately experience a completely different outcome: as we eat, we feel worse, not better. That's because the pleasure and comfort we experience are almost immediately sabotaged by our negative self-judgment. During the very moment we are seeking comfort, we're punishing ourselves. Though the first few bites may very well provide us with a little of what we seek—solace, pleasure, or well-being—that effect quickly dissipates as the judging part of our minds kicks in: *You shouldn't be eating this. There you go again. Can't you deal with anything except by eating?* Instead of giving ourselves permission to experience comfort and pleasure, we go to war with ourselves: *I want to eat this. I shouldn't have it. But I want it. But it's so fattening!*

In addition to the guilt, you might also feel angry at yourself. This is precisely what Kristin Heron, a researcher at Penn State, found when she asked women to keep track of their eating and their moods. The women used handheld computers that asked them several times a day about their moods and eating behaviors. What the research team wanted to know was this: How did mood change as study participants reached for and then ate unhealthy foods such as cookies and chips. What they learned was that so-called junk food didn't comfort diet-conscious participants. Even when participants weren't in a bad mood when they started eating junk food, their moods quickly worsened, especially if they ate large amounts of it.[5]

Mindfulness helps us first become aware of what is really distressing us and then helps us become aware of what can really help. It helps us let go of that rampant self-judgment. It doesn't mean we immediately get rid of those judgmental thoughts and all of that old guilt right away or altogether, but we can begin to loosen its hold on us, until our wiser mind can find a more balanced way of responding.

Other individuals realize that eating urges may be related to dealing with deeper, underlying issues, such as memories of childhood abuse. Something triggers anger—such as an argument with a friend or a spouse—and they find themselves eating uncontrollably. One client had a profound realization as she stood in front of her open fridge in the middle of the night—then took a moment to stop, breathe, and be mindful. "I was about to do my usual binge, and I stopped and realized that I was angry at my husband for something he'd said earlier that day, and angry at my father and at my cousin who had both abused me, but the only person I was hurting was myself. I closed the door and went back to bed."

Sometimes such issues may resolve with mindfulness and more self-care. But if you are struggling with buried pain from the past, deep underlying anger, and/or severe bingeing, it might be best to couple the guidance you find in this book with that of a qualified therapist. Binge eating is often a struggle between eating for comfort and hiding from pain. Some binges get triggered by using food to run away from thoughts or fears. Others begin as a path to self-soothing but very quickly turn into a compulsive urge just to keep eating. Consider that a binge may even be a signal that something troubling has been awakened and is calling to be addressed.

Choosing Comfort Foods

You might assume that you exercise choice every time you eat, because it's convenient, or it's what you want, or it's a healthy option. Quite often, however, we're not fully conscious of why we're making the choice, particularly if we're stressed.

What you reach for when angry, stressed, or sad can date back to your childhood experiences. Your desire to eat may go as far back as your infancy, as your mother fed you when you were crying, and that's normal. It is also likely that one of your favorite comfort foods is something that your parents fed you when you were sad or upset or that was eaten in your household as a special treat or to celebrate. As you got older, you may have found comfort in new foods that friends, coworkers, or coaches offered to you during celebrations. This is why favorite comfort foods vary from person to person. For one person it might be doughnuts. For another, it's vanilla pudding or the warmth of a bowl of soup. For yet another, it's fast food, perhaps reminding you of the hamburgers or fried chicken at family picnics.

No matter what formed the initial association, over time your feelings and this food intertwined. The more tied your emotions become to food, the more automatic your response, causing you to reach for food without even thinking about it. And no low-calorie substitute will do. If you really want chocolate cake but you try to find comfort in low-calorie rice cakes, you'll end up still craving the chocolate cake, and you'll probably just head for it later.

Stress and eating have a complex relationship.[6] It may have to do with comfort, with distracting ourselves, or with masking other feelings.[7] But our research shows that mindfulness can help with that.[8] We're more likely to reach for high-calorie comfort when we're under stress, especially if we're also physically hungry. When stress becomes more chronic, your adrenal glands release a hormone called cortisol, which increases appetite. At the end of the day, we're also tired, so we're not as able to make decisions we'll feel happy about later on. Add a strong emotion to the mix—especially a negative one—and many people reach for the very foods they've told themselves all day long *not* to eat, even grabbing calorie-laden convenience foods that they don't particularly enjoy. Many of us, when we're not hungry, might agree that there's not much available from a vending machine that is both nutritious and tasty. Yet when we're in front of such a machine and it's late afternoon and we're also feeling stressed or anxious, how likely is it that we'll insert a dollar or two and go for the bag of chips or cookies (or both), even ones we don't particularly like?

For many people, it's very likely.

We often feel guilty when we reach for those comfort foods, but this guilt may be unnecessary. You don't feel naughty when you desire other things. For instance, when you are at a social gathering and a friend tells you about the latest and greatest gadget that he or she just purchased, you may consider buying it yourself—without feeling guilty. Instead, you'll reflect (wisely) on that desire: "Do I need it? Do I have enough money for it? Is it worth the price?" If you answer "yes" to those questions, you might go ahead and buy it and feel good about doing so.

Once you become mindfully aware of your desire for food, you'll be able to benefit from what I call the *Power of Choice*, a firm decision—based on inner and outer wisdom—about what and how much to eat. With wisdom as your guide, you'll no longer feel pulled under by the power of food. The power will instead come from your choice of how you'll satisfy your desire for pleasure, comfort, health, and satisfaction. You'll consider how intensely you want particular foods, whether they fit into your health needs, and whether they're worth the caloric price tag. In this way, you'll make an informed decision to eat or not to eat, how much to eat, and what foods to eat. And if you decide to go ahead and eat, you'll enjoy the experience rather than destroying it with guilt and self-doubt.

FAQ

Why are many comfort foods so high in starch, sugar, and/or fat?

It may be because our ancient ancestors often went hungry. Now after years of evolution, our brains are wired to reward us for consuming high-calorie fare. The food industry knows this. Just seeing or smelling high-fat, high-sugar, or high-starch foods causes a brain chemical called dopamine to surge, making us think, "I want that."[9] And then, when we reach for the foods we yearn for, we do really feel better, at least initially, as dopamine rewards us for what we've just eaten. Does this make us addicted? I would argue no. Almost anything pleasurable increases our levels of dopamine. Getting pleasure from food is natural—and normal. Getting out of balance with seeking and experiencing this pleasure is the problem. If we're not in touch with our bodies and minds, we can easily get confused.

Balanced vs. Unbalanced Eating

You may think that the message of this chapter is to eat only when you feel physically hungry and never eat out of desire for pleasure or for comfort. On the contrary, it really can be normal and healthy to eat foods just because you *want* to. Furthermore, it's normal to eat in response to emotions from time to time.

As it turns out, it's not abnormal to eat in response to emotions, both positive and negative, extreme and mild. In formative research I did early on in my career, I found that about 40 percent of the men in our study were relaxed about food, enjoyed snacking, acknowledged occasionally overeating when they were stressed or upset but told us that usually they knew when they'd eaten enough and that they rarely felt guilty about their eating. I call these individuals *Balanced Eaters*. The pattern for the women was striking and concerning: only about 15 percent of the women fit into this balanced eating group because most of the women, if they ate in these ways, felt guilty and then would either vow to go back on their overly restrictive diets or end up eating even more.[10]

That you want delicious food or eat to soothe a bad mood doesn't make you a bad person. In fact, it makes you normal. What's more appropriate to ask yourself is whether your eating is *in balance* or *out of balance*.

Someone who is out of balance goes back and forth between overrestricting and overindulging. *Out-of-Balance Eaters* often have only a very short list of coping strategies to turn to when they're in a bad mood, feeling stressed, had a bad day, or are really angry. For some, there may be only one item on their coping list: food. When they turn to it, they tend to eat a lot, feel guilty about it, overcompensate the following day by "being good," skipping breakfast, and trying to subsist on something light for lunch, and then falling apart in the late afternoon or early evening again due to extreme hunger, fatigue, and cravings—and perhaps more stress. They start nibbling. Soon they're feeling guilty. They go on eating, feeling as if they just couldn't stop. End result, they go to bed feeling full, bloated, and guilty, and they start the cycle over again the following day.

Balanced Eaters, on the other hand, have many different coping strategies to lean on. Sure, food might be one of them, but it's just one part of a rich web of options. They might have ice cream to soothe a sorrow, but they don't undo that comfort by berating themselves with guilt. Then they lean on noncaloric coping strategies. Maybe they call a friend or go for a walk or write in a journal or do something else. They don't keep on eating.

Balanced Eaters also know that food cannot solve their problems. They enjoy the cookie, and then they go to something else.

Forming a healthier relationship with food isn't about banning certain foods from your life. Nor is it about never eating in certain situations, including when you are in need of some comfort. A range of coping strategies is good.[11] Rather it's about this: Shifting from an unbalanced relationship to a balanced one. It's about expanding your list of coping strategies, giving yourself permission to comfort yourself with food from time to time, fitting it into your food energy budget, and deriving true comfort from the food you do eat. It's not as difficult as you might think. The practices in the second half of this book will lead you through how to make this happen.

FAQ

My eating habits are already out of control. If I let myself off the hook by giving myself permission to eat for comfort or pleasure, won't they become even worse?

Consider how permission may help you feel more in control rather than less so, and balance that with how lack of permission is already affecting your eating. Do you gain anything by criticizing yourself? Does self-criticism consistently stop you from eating something that part of you really wants? You may realize how much this self-criticism leads to overeating rather than preventing it. Every time you criticize yourself, you strengthen the urge to eat as an escape from the pain of the criticism. When you shift from self-criticism to awareness, you still have accountability. Self-acceptance doesn't mean that you don't figure out how to do something different the next time; it means that you don't respond with automatic critical self-judgment that shuts out wisdom. Mindfulness provides a way of being aware and accountable without being judgmental. Cultivating mindfulness has the power to help you let go of old patterns, rather than reinforcing them over and over again.

How You'll Balance Physical Hunger with Desire

There's so much value in tuning in, noticing what's triggering you, and becoming aware of the choices you are making around food. Mindful awareness teaches you how to ask good questions: Am I physically hungry? When did I last eat? Is this a food that I enjoy? How strong is my craving for this? Why? Might I feel satisfied with just a small amount? Have I had enough?

This stopping and checking in is sometimes all it takes for our desire to go from "I must eat that right now" to "I'll have some, but perhaps just a taste." And mean it.

It's important to become aware of these feelings, so you can know why you are eating. The more you cultivate awareness of your level of physical hunger as well as all of the other reasons you want to eat, the more confident you'll be in making decisions about your eating and the better you'll be able to balance your physical need for food with the other reasons you want to eat.

Some theories of obesity suggest that many individuals aren't able to tune in to their inner physical hunger signals in a useful way. But, in my experience, that is rare. I've worked with people who have struggled with their weight for years and who were binge eating almost every day. After just one week of practicing mindful awareness of hunger, some are able to report, with surprise, that for the first time it had been fairly easy to notice how physically hungry they were. After several weeks, they become more confident that they can even distinguish between feeling anxious and feeling truly physically hungry. They might realize that they don't really want the cookies that someone had brought into the office, given they've just had lunch. At another time, they realize that they do want the cookies. It's 10:30 a.m., they had a modest breakfast at 6:30, and they really are physically hungry. Helping themselves to that treat makes sense, and they enjoy it without their usual guilt.

But is this true for everyone? No, it isn't. Some people find it harder, for example, to tune in to feelings of physical hunger but easier to tune in to feelings of physical fullness, which you'll learn about in the next chapter. Everyone is different, and as you explore the mindful eating principles in *The Joy of Half a Cookie*, you'll find that some seem easier to work with than do others.

No matter what resonates in the beginning, eventually the mindfulness tools will come together, allowing you to gain much more freedom over your food environment. Right now, you might rightly feel that you can't have any tempting snack foods at home or at your office. You doubt you'd be able to stop from eating most of the box or bag and, even if you managed to resist, you wouldn't be able to stop thinking about them.

Over time, as you cultivate mindful awareness of your triggers, this will change. At first, it might be subtle. Maybe you can have such foods around, but they must be stored out of sight. With more practice, it might be okay for them to be more accessible as long as you make a mental note: "That's for tomorrow."

As you cultivate mindfulness even more, you may even find that you forget such snacks are there at all. Maybe, one day, much as one of my clients did, you'll open a drawer and find the pack of chips and think, "When did I put that in there?"

And in that moment, you'll realize that those so-called problem foods have stopped being a problem for you.

Try This Now

I've taught hunger awareness to countless people, and most of them have picked it up very quickly. You might even find yourself getting acquainted with your physical hunger right now. What sensations of physical hunger do you notice? Where do you feel them? If you rated them on a 1 to 10 scale, with 1 = "no hunger" and 10 = "starving," how intense are they? How are these feelings of physical hunger different from other feelings, like anxiety, boredom, or loneliness? Or craving a particular food? What if you rate craving the same way, perhaps with "mild desire" at the low end and "can't stop thinking about it" at the high end? And how does that feel different from real physical hunger? We'll be spending more time on tuning in to this type of self-awareness in the second half of this book, but this can get you started!

CHAPTER FOUR

Full of Food, Empty of Satisfaction

What Leads You to the Next Bite

In the previous chapter, you learned that we often start eating without much awareness. Just as common is staying on autopilot as we continue to eat well past the point of satisfaction and comfort.

When is "enough" truly enough?

Maybe we're socializing with friends. Maybe we're reading a book, working away at our computers, or watching a movie. Or maybe our minds are just wandering. End result: We take bite after bite, but we derive little if any true pleasure, often just eating until the food is gone. Even if we've just consumed a delicious meal, we're left with a lack of satisfaction. Where did all the food go? And when?

In addition to this sense of mild dissatisfaction, there may be physical discomfort. We might have to undo the top button on our pants or uncinch our belt to make room. Or we feel bloated, sluggish, dull, and in need of a nap.

We've all experienced these sensations, and without mindfulness, it can seem as if there were not much we could do to prevent them, that we will always lack willpower or self-control when facing certain foods or situations. There is, however, a way to gain freedom. What's really going on when we overeat is this: We're out of touch with the internal cues to stop eating—with our taste buds as they lose sensitivity, with the growing sense of distension in our stomachs, and with changes in our overall sense of well-being. At the same time, we're also overly influenced by external triggers to continue eating, ranging from seeing the food on our plate to the waitress offering another bottomless basket of fries, more bread, or the dessert special.

The Elements of Enough

When I ask people about how they know when to stop eating, the most common answer is: "Well, it takes 20 minutes." One problem is that you can eat a lot of food in 20 minutes! However, the good news is that "it takes 20 minutes" is only partially true.

Our bodies do tell us when to stop eating, but they send us these signals much earlier than 20 minutes. The problem is that, when we eat mindlessly, we often miss the cues. The signals are there; they just escape our notice, much the same way we might not hear our spouse tell us something if we're reading or watching television. Only when someone raises his or her voice do we take notice. It's the same with our sense of "enough." When we're not paying attention, we don't notice its presence. Then, as we become uncomfortably full, we suddenly think, "Why did I eat so much?"

To feel satisfied sooner, we need only listen to the messages our bodies send. As you eat, three different processes are taking place that work together to create a sensation of "enough." The three elements include the immediate response of our taste buds and our sense of *taste satisfaction*; a growing sense of *stomach fullness*, which depends on the volume of what we've eaten; and increasing *body satiety*, which is related to a rise in blood sugar and other nutrients as they are absorbed into our bodies from what we've eaten.[1]

Let's take a closer look at these three processes, starting with something that happens with your very first bite of food: taste satisfaction.

TASTE SATISFACTION

Some foods taste better than other foods. We all know this—and we know that our preference for certain foods may be different from other peoples' preferences. *Taste satisfaction* is the term I use both for how good a food tastes in general and how it tastes in the moment.

Foods taste better when we're hungry and in need of calories because our taste buds light up brighter, bringing their message strongly up to our brains. As we continue eating, taste buds become tired rather quickly—more rapidly if we are less hungry and more slowly if we are very hungry, so food also tastes better toward the beginning of a meal than toward the end.

Our taste buds can detect five types of signals—sweet, sour, bitter, salty, and umami (the Japanese word for savory or protein-type tastes). So your sensation of flavor can go up and down over the course of a meal as different flavors reawaken different taste responses. Still, no matter how pleasant a food might be initially, our taste buds are capable of experiencing and registering flavors fully for only a short period of time. Once taste buds tire, eating more of the same food won't restimulate them. The flavor sensation may be reawakened when switching to a different food, and then that type of taste sensitivity will weaken. You might come back later in the meal to that first food and get more of the flavor back, as your tastes buds recover somewhat, but you won't be as hungry as before, so that will also lessen the taste experience.

When our taste buds lose their sensitivity to the flavor of a food, I call this *taste satiety* (technically referred to as *sensory-specific satiety*), causing taste satisfaction to drop. It's useful to think of taste satisfaction from 10 (incredible) down to 1 (yuck). But rather than a straight line, like hunger, think of it as a meter that can fluctuate back and forth a little, as depicted on page 56. It may go up for the first few bites, especially for more complex foods, as we fully savor the experience. But if you carefully pay attention, you may be surprised to find how quickly taste satiety begins to set in, and taste satisfaction begins to drop. Then, if you give your taste buds some time to recover while you eat a different food, it may go back up again, but not as far as it did when you were hungrier. Taste satisfaction then gradually moves down even more, often dropping down a lot at about a typical serving amount (but this varies by person, the type of food, and your hunger level—experiment for yourself!).

Of the three internal satiety or eating satisfaction cues, taste satiety is the swiftest. It's for this reason that paying attention to moment-to-moment changes in taste satisfaction is so powerful, but most of us just aren't aware at all. So we don't pay attention, and we may even *chase the flavor*, continually eating to try to recapture the pleasure of the first few bites, which is impossible. We just keep eating, thinking "I want more . . . I want more . . . I want more," when, in reality, we're getting less satisfaction or true pleasure. This experience can also fuel that sense of feeling addicted or of being out of control around certain foods.

Without awareness, you might chase after the initial flavor of a dessert or the potato flavor of a chip. With mindful awareness, however, you'll quickly find that salty, fatty, and sweet foods tend to satisfy—and then overwhelm—your taste buds relatively quickly, and *all* you might be left with is the sweetness or the saltiness or the greasiness. Many of my clients tell me, for example, that they can't even find an underlying flavor in most potato chips. All they taste is salt. While the first bite of sweet, salty, or fatty foods might taste amazing—hitting the perfect 10 in terms of flavor—that appeal quickly wears off. After just a few bites, the majority of foods that most people sort into the "too tempting to even think about eating" category actually offer most people very little enjoyment. And the more processed and less gourmet the food, the less flavor you are likely to noticc.

You might also be chasing the memory of a flavor: eating to recapture an experience you had years ago when eating a similar food. It's indeed true that our memories are powerful, and they *will* kick in. That commercial processed chocolate chip cookie really does taste better if your memory reminds you of all the really good homemade ones you had as a child. So tuning in mindfully to your taste experience can help you to decide whether it's worthwhile to eat this particular cookie right now. Perhaps, it might be better to occasionally treat yourself to a bakery chocolate chip cookie and fully enjoy it, even saving the other half for later to enjoy all over again.

Or you may notice that your taste meter isn't going very high at all: your taste buds are telling you that this food isn't very good. And then it can tell you when to stop eating something fantastic because the taste meter has dropped too much to make it worthwhile to eat more; better to save the rest for later! And both of these can happen after only a few bites. So rather than super-sizing something for satisfaction, you might want to consider *mini-sizing* it: You maximize the pleasure and minimize the calories.

This kind of awareness allows you to cultivate your *inner gourmet*: choosing the flavor-rich foods you love. When you cultivate your inner gourmet, you'll consider whether you will enjoy that bowl of ice cream a lot, a little, or not at all. Perhaps if it's your favorite flavor—such as Ben & Jerry's Cherry Garcia is for me—you'll know that you're about to enjoy it a lot, as you savor every bite of the experience. You'll do this fearlessly, knowing that your taste buds will call "enough" long before the pint is empty, and that the pint will last the whole week or more.

On the other hand, let's say it's not your favorite ice cream. Maybe it's even been left too long in the freezer. You might have a bite just to check. The bite confirms your suspicions—it's really past its prime. So you toss the whole container, saving those calories for something more special.

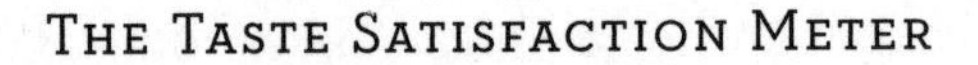

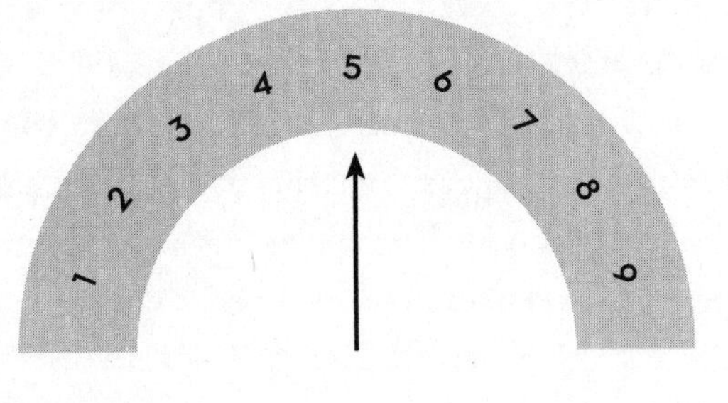

Try This Now

The next time you are eating, pick one food to pay particular attention to. It's easier if it's a simple food, rather than one with many mixed-in flavors. In Part Two, I'll be sharing several practices to help you cultivate your inner gourmet, but this is a way to get started. Notice how much taste occurs in the first bite. The taste may be subtle but enjoyable, or intense but not so good. So it's a combination of the two. That's how high the taste satisfaction meter is going, perhaps to an 8? Then take another small amount. How is the taste changing? Is your enjoyment going up? To a 9? Or down? At what point does the flavor start to drop off? How about the third bite? And the fourth? Perhaps to a 5, and then to a 3. You can keep on eating it, of course, and see how the taste continues to change. Tune in to your experiences, how they compare in the moment to other times you've eaten this food or to memories that may come from long ago.

STOMACH FULLNESS

Tuning in to taste satisfaction can help you feel satisfied throughout your meal, as you notice the point when it drops for each food you are eating. But noticing stomach fullness can help you know when to finish the meal. Stomach fullness is what you feel in and around your stomach based on the weight and volume of what you've eaten. As more and more food goes into your stomach, you'll notice a growing sense of distension or fullness, as your stomach swells, stimulating nearby nerves. It is not just the opposite of hunger, as different physiological processes are involved.

The sensation of fullness varies tremendously by type of food you've eaten. Some foods and beverages fill you up quickly, perhaps within just a few minutes, but don't keep you feeling full for very long. Other foods—such as heavy, fibrous, water-dense foods like bean dishes, fruit, and salad—also fill you up quickly and the sensation of fullness will last longer. There are all sorts of other variations.

Similar to physical hunger, it's helpful to tune in to stomach fullness by using a 1 to 10 *fullness scale*, with 1 being "empty" and 10 being "as full as you can imagine" (post-Thanksgiving dinner or post-binge). Many of the people I've worked with are surprised at how easily they could tune in to these feelings once they began to observe them mindfully during a meal. But clients who are heavier or who binge eat come back to the next group session exclaiming that they often end up eating to a 13 or 15! Others come back realizing how distinct fullness is from hunger; you can be a little bit full and still be somewhat hungry. But all begin to explore the feelings of "enough."

Much as our experience of taste and flavor is affected by memories and past experiences, so is our understanding of what is a right amount of fullness. For many people, it may seem all or nothing. Before learning how to be more mindful, many of my workshop participants assumed there was only one kind of fullness: stuffed. They realize that the message they got growing up was the more, the better. Perhaps they came from a family that, at times, didn't have enough food (what we now call *food insecurity*). Or they grew up with the message that super-sizing it, whether at the dinner table or at a fast-food place, was always better.[2]

As they become mindfully aware of their fullness sensations, they understand that they can enjoy many different levels of fullness. They begin to recognize that moderate levels of fullness are indeed far more comfortable. They also learn that they can adjust their fullness goal, depending on their plans right after eating. For example, perhaps they're planning to exercise in an hour, but they're hungry. So they choose an energy bar instead of a full meal to take the edge off their hunger but without feeling uncomfortably full. Then there are holidays, splurges, and special occasions when going to a high degree of fullness—an 8, 9, or 10—might be fine, even if somewhat uncomfortable. Despite popular belief, it's really okay and quite normal a few times a year, to look forward to feeling stuffed. Many people who are thin and in good balance with their eating do this without feeling guilty about it. They know they will enjoy the few times a year that they will consume seconds or thirds, plus desserts and then put up with the related discomfort.

With more awareness, you may realize that continuing to eat, whether at a meal or out of the cupboard, often has to do with other issues beyond the desire to feel full. There's the social pressure of the group, of wanting to be part of the party, or of giving in—over and over again—to encouragement to just have some more. Or you might become aware that you are using eating and food to fend off boredom or other feelings or to express your rebellious self.

Noticing these habitual thoughts and habits can help you tune in to how you make judgments about how much food is the right amount. And there really is no single right answer. A light snack makes sense if you will have a regular meal in an hour or two; a heavier lunch may make sense if you know you'll be working through to dinnertime.

As you tune in to stomach fullness, you'll be able to better sense your developing fullness after every few bites, so you can finish your meals feeling just right rather than uncomfortably full. Over time, you'll also learn how certain foods affect your sensations of fullness for the better or the worse. This information will enable you to make wiser decisions about what foods to eat, when to eat them, and when to stop.

Try This Now

To see how quickly you can tune in to stomach fullness, start to pay attention to the changing sensations as you eat. When do you start to feel a growing sense of fullness? When does that sense of fullness change into discomfort? Play with these experiences, and realize that you have a choice in how full you get at every meal and every time you eat.

HOW DIETING DISCONNECTS US FROM "ENOUGH"

There's nothing wrong with you for being out of touch with the elements of "enough." It's not a character flaw. Nor is it a sign of weakness. It's only that no one has taught you to listen to your body in this way. If anything, you've been taught the opposite: to ignore your internal signals to stop eating. Most younger children, research shows, are in touch with their sensations of fullness, and they tend to leave food on their plates quite easily. If you are a parent, then maybe you've seen this for yourself. Perhaps you've given your young child a heaping serving of ice cream and were amazed when, a short time later, your son or daughter said, "I'm full" and walked away from the table, even though some of the ice cream remained to be eaten.

As children age, however, this natural connection weakens. In part, this might be due to conditioning as the well-meaning adults in their lives encourage them to clean their plates and to never waste food.[3] It also might stem from distracted eating. Perhaps, in your home, dinner took place with a television blaring in front of you or in the background. Or maybe you often ate on the go, while rushing from one task to another. When we're distracted, it's hard to tune in to our body's signals to stop eating.

Here's something else that can make it more difficult to know when to stop eating after you've consumed a reasonable amount: dieting.

Most diets impose external, artificial limits on what and how much you can eat, and this can shift you even further away from your ability to self-regulate how much you eat. Diets define how much you are *allowed* to eat in order to stay on the diet, causing you to shift into a willpower or self-control mind-set. This is appealing for some, in part because it reduces the number of decisions you must make in a day. Rather than deciding for yourself how much to eat and when to eat it, the diet decides for you, and you attempt to make yourself follow what the diet says.

The problem, though, is that these plans don't take into account how much food you really need to feel full and satisfied. If you end a meal feeling unsatisfied, you learn to do one of two things (or possibly both). You might distract yourself and disconnect from these internal sensations. Or, if your eating plan allows it, you might fill up on "free" foods. These free foods—such as cucumbers, carrots, and celery—are extremely low in calories, rich in water, and high in volume. Such foods come with a low caloric price tag and take up a lot of space in the stomach, meeting that perceived need to feel really full.

But whether you are eating overly large portions of something rich in calories like french fries or overly large portions of a free food like carrots, you are still eating overly large portions to fill your stomach. And you're probably eating them mindlessly. As you eat to fill your stomach, you disconnect even more from the useful information your body is giving you, and you continue to perceive very full as a desirable state.

Dieting also disconnects you from taste awareness and taste satisfaction. You're not directed to choose foods that help you find your inner gourmet or be truly satisfied with a smaller serving of granola for breakfast, a little bit of rich sauce on that 4-ounce piece of steak or fish for dinner, or small amounts of your favorite ice cream for a snack. Further, overeating a free food is virtually guaranteed to take you past the point of actually enjoying the taste or flavor of it, reinforcing the habit of quantity over quality.

Rather than disconnecting from taste and fullness by following a diet and losing 10 or 20 or more pounds as quickly as possible, it's much more beneficial in the long term to cultivate the ability to tune in to your sense of "enough" and to recognize the common triggers that tend to trip you up.

BODY SATIETY

There is one more important signal. As your body digests your meal and food nutrients enter your bloodstream, blood sugar rises and levels of various biochemicals change. This initially increases your sense of energy and well-being, but then decreases again if you overeat. As with stomach fullness, body satiety doesn't take 20 minutes to start to kick in, either.

Body satiety starts to set in a few minutes after your first bite. The truth to the "it takes 20 minutes" guideline is that body satiety may reach its peak or plateau about 20 minutes after your last bite of food, depending on the type of food and how much you've eaten. A soda or a glass of juice, where the sugar energy is quickly absorbed, may hit its peak sooner, but leave you feeling satisfied for only a short period of time. A healthy power bar with complex carbohydrates and about the same number of calories will start to be absorbed relatively quickly but will last longer. Even longer lasting would be a combination of complex carbohydrates and protein, with more calories and more bulk. Two different lunches with the same amount of food energy might leave you feeling sated for very different lengths of time, depending on the nutrient components.[4]

Body satiety, therefore, doesn't lend itself as well to using the 10-point scale or meter that applied to hunger, taste, and fullness, and isn't that useful in knowing when to end a meal. But tuning in to it can be very valuable in learning to trust decisions about what to eat and when to stop eating, in order to keep yourself from overeating a larger meal, and in recognizing that even a small amount of food is bringing valuable food energy into your body.

The Paradox of Overeating

You may have heard advice cautioning you to avoid doing certain things while you eat because they will *cause* you to overeat: eating too fast, lingering at the table for too much time, eating with other people, and so on. Interestingly, whether you overeat has much more to do with how you eat—mindlessly versus mindfully—than with any of these external factors.

For instance, consider the paradox of ever-present food. It's often thought that the longer you sit with food in front of you, the more you'll eat, especially if you are sitting with people who are still eating. This is why many of us tend to overeat at parties. We're around food for many, many hours.[5] But spending longer at the table doesn't *have* to translate into eating more. When Paul Rozin, a psychologist at the University of Pennsylvania, studied the differences between how the French eat and how Americans eat, he found that the French stayed *longer* at meals than do Americans, even though they eat *less*.[6] How can this be? As it turns out, the French tend to eat much more mindfully. As Mireille Guiliano explained in *French Women Don't Get Fat*, they opt for rich foods they know they will enjoy, and then they savor those foods, soaking up each mouthful of flavor.[7] They are masters at cultivating the inner gourmet, and we can learn from their example.

Food variety offers yet another paradox. The more choices we're offered (chicken, broccoli, bread, potatoes, and a dessert versus just chicken and broccoli) and the more complex a food (mint chocolate chip cookies with M&M's versus butter cookies), the more we might eat, if we are eating mindlessly. For example, when Barbara Rolls and her team offered study participants sandwiches with four distinct fillings, the participants consumed about 30 percent more food than those who were offered sandwiches with just one type of filling.[8] Does this mean that you should always consume simple foods and limit your choices? No, not at all. It only shows why it's so important to remain aware of your sense of hunger, taste, and fullness. When I've shown people how to do this, they've been able to navigate environments with lots of variety and find they eat less rather than more.

Mindfulness can make the difference between saying "Enough!" instead of "Might as well keep on eating" in the face of external triggers such as the following:

- **Super-sized portions:** If we're eating mindlessly, the larger a portion of food is, the more of that food we'll eat, even if we don't like it. If we're eating mindfully, the portions don't have as much pull.
- **Financial pressure:** We often eat more if it's a bargain. Even the timing of when we pay our bill matters, as Israeli researchers have found. When diners paid before they sat down at an all-you-can-eat sushi restaurant, they consumed 4.5 more units of sushi than if they paid afterward.[9] Again, this is true only if we are not tuned in to what we are doing.
- **Social pressure:** How often do you eat that roll in the bread basket—that you're not even enjoying—just because it's there and everyone else is?

This is the beginning of a list, and you may notice some other triggers that would go on it for you. Perhaps eating with certain friends or family members or in a particular setting makes it harder to tune in to and limit what you eat to the right amount. As you become mindfully aware of the physiological, psychological, social, and environmental triggers that encourage you to keep eating, you'll gain perspective and wisdom. And when you pair that wisdom with awareness of your internal cues to stop eating, you'll gain true freedom.

FAQ

I've heard that I should eat slowly by putting down my fork between each bite, and counting the numbers of bites, even up to 100 per mouthful. Is this something that you recommend?

While eating slowly is a worthy goal, it can also be quite difficult to put into practice. When I counsel clients who are struggling with their weight, they may tell me that they've tried to put their fork down between bites, chew thoroughly, or slow their pace way down, but that it all feels mechanical. The obsessive focus on continually putting down their forks distracts them from enjoying their food. They're counting bites, instead of enjoying them. When you become mindfully aware of the sensations of taste satisfaction and fullness, you'll be able to stop eating sooner, and you'll feel *more* satisfied.

"I've Blown It," and Other Thoughts That Get Us into Trouble

In the previous chapter, you learned of several types of thoughts that help us justify that first bite. Many other thoughts can also justify eating out of control and are therefore pretty self-defeating. Sometimes these are referred to as "distorted thinking": patterns of thoughts that become habits, but are not really accurate, nor particularly helpful. Let's explore some of the most common ones in relation to eating.

I have to clean my plate! Nearly all of us have said this to ourselves at some point. At the same time, this kind of mindless thinking isn't logical. There's no relationship between how much you eat and whether children somewhere else in the world are starving. And if you are eating food you don't enjoy and energy your body doesn't need, then you're still wasting food. It would be much less of a waste to set aside what you can't finish now so you can enjoy it later, when your taste buds are fresh and you are hungry again. Consider this: As you gradually reduce how much you (and perhaps your family) are eating, you can also reduce your grocery bills. And you can consider contributing the difference to a charity that really will help feed others who desperately need the food.

I've blown it! What's the "I've Blown It" effect? It's when your negative, controlling inner parent ("You shouldn't have it") is bouncing off your willful inner child ("But I want it"). Eventually, you end up with "I've blown it" followed by "I might as well keep going," "Here I go again," or something similar. The "I've Blown It" effect, as I phrase it, was identified in the 1970s by Alan Marlatt, the late director of the Addictive Behaviors Research Center at the University of Washington, whose technical term for it was the *abstinence violation effect.* He found that recovering addicts who considered a single slip up, such as smoking one cigarette or drinking one beer, as evidence of their innate lack of willpower were more likely to completely relapse than those who saw it for what it was: Just one slipup.[10]

This is also true with food. Scientists have been studying such patterns in food intake for some time, showing that chronic dieters are also susceptible to the "I've Blown It" effect. One study started off by asking participants to consume zero, one, or two large milk-shakes, and then offered them different flavors of ice cream to taste.[11] Nondieters ate progressively less ice cream as the milkshakes got larger. The good news was that dieters also ate less after the very large, 30-ounce shake, but ate more ice cream after the 16-ounce shake. This suggests that while dieters, at least those in this study, could be responsive to very high levels of satiety, they would stray from their diet intentions when the violation was more moderate.

If you tell yourself that you've blown it, then you'll probably go on to do just that. If, on the other hand, you keep a balanced sense of perspective and tell yourself "Oh, well, maybe I ate too much, but next time I'll be more mindful," then you'll understand that there's no such thing as "blowing it." Right now, it might feel as if you go from "I want to eat that" to "I've blown it" as just one part of an uncontrollable cycle or chain reaction. With mindfulness, you can stop the chain reaction at any point. Every moment is an opportunity to be mindfully aware of your ability to stop, pause, and head in a different direction.

I want to get my money's worth! This one often comes up at all-you-can-eat buffets, and when we're served bottomless beverages, fries, and other dishes. Even after eating to an uncomfortable point of fullness, you might think, "I'm going to make one more trip so I can get my money's worth." This is irrational because you pay the same amount for the meal, no matter how much you eat. End result, you gain weight on the scale, but your bank balance remains pretty much the same.

Mindfulness doesn't mean that you push these thoughts out of your mind (you probably wouldn't be able to at first) or never follow what your thoughts suggest. It's about paying attention to them and making conscious, rather than automatic choices, by responding rather than reacting. You'll be able to see these thoughts as "just thoughts," rather than inner commands. For instance, if you're eating out and the dessert cart comes by, you'll consider: Is there one offered that you will really enjoy? How full are you already? If you continue to eat, how will it affect your day's food balance? Perhaps you're not that full, you've eaten lightly earlier in the day, and one of the desserts is your favorite—so let yourself enjoy! But if the opposite is true, you have the power to decide to let it go.

By considering such questions, you'll be able to arrive at a firm, guilt-free decision to continue to eat or not to, and you'll be aware of the decisions you are making. Your eating will become a conscious choice, and you'll be able to enjoy the experience even as you are losing weight.

Finding Your Inner Gourmet

Mindfulness acts as a counterpoint against the lure of external triggers. It helps you become more aware of all of the processes that add up to feeling you've had enough. Use this awareness to inform your choice of when to stop eating, whether it's a snack or a meal or a particular food, and you'll no longer have to rely on willpower or policing yourself.

Instead you'll make your choices based on what you want and what you enjoy. Rather than forcing yourself to eat low-fat or low-carb foods you truly don't enjoy, you'll feel confident about making a completely different and liberating choice: savoring small amounts of the foods that call to you the most. You'll cultivate your inner gourmet. You'll go for just a few fried chips rather than the baked ones (if that's what you prefer) or for the homemade brownie rather than the low-sugar one that came from the store. You might even become the thinner picky eater, relishing some of those healthier foods, in your family! But out of a place of pleasure, healthy self-constraint, and self-care rather than fear and anxiety.

On the other hand, you might even find, as so many of my workshop participants have, that some foods that you once thought of as tempting or dangerous stop calling to you altogether. Before learning how to eat mindfully, one of my clients, for example, believed that she *loved* a certain brand of shortbread cookie: Lorna Doones. For years, she'd taken these to potlucks and office parties, and she even used them to make her pie crusts. She told us she was known at her work as the Lorna Doone Lady.

Yet when, during a session, she ate two of these cookies mindfully, she was shocked and somewhat dismayed. "I don't even like this cookie!" she exclaimed. "It's too salty, too dry, and after the first one, I couldn't even taste the flavor."

This can be your experience, too. Or not. Someone else in the group had never eaten them before, and discovered she rather liked them, but was satisfied with just 3 or 4.

CHAPTER FIVE

Cultivating Outer Wisdom

The Knowledge That Will Set You Free

In the past several chapters, I've shared how inner wisdom—using awareness of hunger, of satisfaction, of emotions, of thoughts—can help you end the struggle over when to eat and how much to eat. By cultivating inner wisdom, you may find that you naturally eat less and, consequently, lose weight.

But, as I learned when developing MB-EAT, inner wisdom alone may not be enough. Initially, when I taught this approach, we talked about the need to consider nutrition, decrease calories, and increase activity in order to manage weight, but I did not include mindfulness practices that involved engaging these issues systematically and from a different approach than do more traditional diet programs. Our data showed about a third of our study participants lost weight using inner wisdom practices alone, but others lost little to no weight at all, and others *gained* weight.

Though the best predictor of success was how much mindfulness practice, both sitting meditation and mini-meditations people told us they were using, several other patterns appeared. Most people could tune in to the pleasure from small amounts of their favorite calorically dense foods, like ice cream, but some would ignore fullness signals and eat larger amounts of foods that they saw as healthier, such as granola or nuts, and those foods can still add up to lots of calories. Other participants told me they could sometimes eat smaller amounts of tempting foods, but would overeat at times due to social pressure or other stressors. Some other individuals were no longer eating out of control but became grazers, spreading their calories out during the day. They had taken in the message that, as long as they weren't overeating, they could still go to food for other reasons. Regardless, many were not taking into account that if they wanted to lose weight, the only option was to create new day-to-day patterns of eating less food that they could sustain indefinitely into the future.

As I reflected on these results, we decided to start teaching participants to mindfully consider calories as simply *information about food energy*. I also realized that I could do the same with other elements of outer wisdom, including nutrition and physical activity. And once I incorporated these important practices into MB-EAT, the success of the participants dramatically improved—and in our last program, no one gained weight.

Embracing the C-Word

The word *calories* has become so psychologically linked with the struggle over eating that it makes many people feel anxious. But knowledge of calories—what I call food energy—can be just as liberating as knowledge of anything else that you might fear. As a psychologist, I've worked with many people with anxiety about other things in their lives, from fear of snakes to fear of flying to fear of open spaces (agoraphobia). The answer for dealing with these fears is not to avoid them but to gradually learn to become more relaxed, more open to experiencing them in new ways, and finally to see them just as they are. Most snakes aren't poisonous, most people fly safely, and open spaces aren't really dangerous. Gradually learning to consider calories just as information really can be much more empowering than looking the other way, or alternatively, counting obsessively.

By embracing this knowledge about food in a mindful way, you'll make more informed decisions around eating. Consider what might happen if you never looked at price tags while you were out shopping. Even if you were careful to purchase only what you truly needed—one pair of shoes rather than three, for instance—you might still spend more money than you earn, especially if that pair of shoes costs $100 when you have only $50.

Similarly, it's hard to tell just by glancing at a pair of shoes how much they might cost. You might think that they're within your budget. Then, when you check the price tag, you might be surprised. And just like everyone's financial budget, we all have a food energy budget, but how this is set is quite complex and affected by many factors, including our metabolism, activity level, and our weight. Even the scientists don't agree exactly.[1]

I'm often asked, "How many calories do I actually need each day?" This is hard to predict as it varies substantially, as everyone is different, and it may vary as much as from 10 to 15 calories for every pound we weigh, every day, to maintain itself. This is quite a wide range, if you think about it. For example, for someone who weighs 150 pounds, that translates into a range from 1,500 calories to 2,250 calories per day, with about 1,800 in the middle. Other estimates place the average amount needed between 2,000 and 2,400 calories per day. Someone at the lower end may have a slower metabolism (they burn food energy more efficiently) and be less active (physical exercise not only burns more calories, but also increases metabolism for several hours). And someone at the higher end may be much more active, with a higher metabolism. This range doesn't include even lower levels for a very sedentary person or higher levels for the serious athlete. So as weight increases, perhaps to about 200 pounds, the range could be anywhere from about 2,000 calories to over 3,000 calories per day, with about 2,500 in the middle to maintain that weight.

Another way to think about budgeting your food energy intake is to consider that 1,800–2,000 calories works out to about 100 calories of food energy per waking hour, with some left over for sleep time. This, of course, will depend on your weight, activity level, and metabolism, but it's a rule-of-thumb our participants have found very helpful in estimating what they might need to eat to get through to their next meal without getting overly hungry and without undue worry about overeating.

Many popular diets pick a number for you, often about 1,200 calories. But if your calorie need is much higher, you may feel unnecessarily ravenous on such a plan. Yes, you'd lose weight quickly, but not without significant hunger, light-headedness, and frequent cravings. In addition, while you'd know how to eat the way the diet requires, you wouldn't know how to eat at your new dietary maintenance goal level of perhaps 1,800, 2,000, or 2,200 calories.

Even if you did know your goal number for sure—based on your metabolism and level of physical activity—it's not realistic or even necessary to expect yourself to consume the same number of calories every single day. Holding yourself to inflexible rules (only 400 calories per meal, for example) will lead to your inner child eventually rebelling, triggering some of the distorted thinking described in Chapter 3. It also doesn't teach you how to be both flexible and balanced.

You really can consume 2,000 calories some days and 1,400 other days and still lose weight. Just like budgeting, you don't have to spend the same amount every day. But, to lose weight, it has to average out over every few days to fewer calories than your body needs at your current weight. And in the long run, it needs to average out to what your body would need for your longer-term goal weight.

So you may be wondering, How do I possibly find the right amount to aim for to lose weight? It's a lot simpler than you may think. All you need to do is this: Eat less than you are currently eating. In my workshops and studies, I never tell participants to eat only a predetermined number of daily calories, but I do encourage them to look for opportunities to remove up to 500 daily calories from what they are currently eating. This is called the *500-Calorie Challenge*. Over a week's time, those daily opportunities to cut 500 calories equal 3,500 fewer calories per week. Again, depending on your activity, metabolism, and genetics, that will lead to a weight loss of 2 to 4 pounds per month, more initially and somewhat less over time as your body adjusts. But it is a good way to begin, particularly if you are heavy, with 50 pounds or more to lose. If you have less to lose, you can consider adjusting this amount downward (for example, by 100 calories for each 10 pounds less). When you hit a plateau, you can consider decreasing by more.

You might choose to have one egg at breakfast rather than two, to use less mayonnaise on a sandwich, and consume a smaller piece of steak at dinner, with less butter on the potato, and half your usual dessert. That adds up to 500 calories (or more). But it's not a rigid diet approach, and these are the kinds of changes you could keep on doing indefinitely. Otherwise, what's the point?

For example, a physician I worked with was puzzled that she had put on about 30 pounds in three years. She then realized, when she checked the box label and measured what she put into her cereal bowl, that her seemingly healthy breakfast consisted of not one but three servings of granola, or over 600 calories. Her quick snacks of two to three energy bars during the day added up to more than 400 calories. Including her regular lunch, dinner, and light evening snack, she was averaging over 2,500 calories per day. The energy bars had served her well during her medical training, when she might not have time to eat, but were no longer a very helpful part of her eating plan. She figured out that she was eating about 500 to 600 more calories than she really needed. She also realized that while she rarely ate until she was too full, she would often reach in her pocket for a granola bar when she wasn't really physically hungry. So she began to look for ways to mindfully take out the extra calories. She decreased her breakfast by about a third and stopped keeping granola bars in her pocket, but she knew she would still eat them on occasion. So she also looked for a couple of other options and the weight began to come off.

When you are mindfully aware of the energy value of different foods as well as the food energy your body needs, you can combine inner wisdom with outer wisdom to make more informed choices about what and how much to eat, and how much—on average—you might need to cut back, without counting every calorie. And you can find ways to do so that you can stay with indefinitely. One participant put an even more positive spin on it: "I think of it as calories I *get* to spend—and 2,200 calories per day, on average, actually sounds like quite a bit. I'm not dieting—I'm enjoying!"

And it has become much easier to find out the caloric value of most foods, whether from the labels on the back of packages, online lists, or new requirements for chain restaurants to make available the number of calories in most of their offerings. Again, you just need to take a few relaxing breaths, check in, and see calories as information that's comparable to the price tags on items at your local store.

You are managing your calorie budget in the same way as any other expense, rather than becoming anxious about it.

Moving Beyond Food as Poison

Of course, healthy eating is about more than just calories. Some foods (vegetables, fruits, legumes, beans, whole grains, lean meats) are generally more filling and certainly more nutritious than other foods (soft drinks, highly processed snack chips, sugar-and-fat rich desserts, and highly processed meats). In the past several years, we've all seen the headlines about the damaging health effects of refined sugars, salt, and certain types of fat. You won't find a nutrition expert in the country who will tell you that soft drinks and Cheez Doodles are healthy, and I won't tell you that either. At the same time, however, this doesn't mean that you can't eat these foods occasionally or in small amounts. They are not poison. It only means you have to find the right balance.

And that balance varies from person to person. Based on your age and health, you may decide to eat more or less sugar, salt, and fat than someone else. For instance, if you have diabetes or are at risk for it, you'll probably opt for far fewer sweets than someone who doesn't have this health condition. If you have high blood pressure, then you'll consume less sodium. It's the same with heart disease and many other conditions.

Instead of a good food/bad food approach, you might consider adopting an eat more/eat less approach. Eat more of the foods that contribute to good health and fewer of the ones that don't. And look for ways to find a balance. As you inform yourself about nutrition, you may find, for instance, that you can lightly salt vegetables if you simultaneously cut back on processed or canned foods, generally very high in sodium. Also, as you develop your inner wisdom, you may find that you prefer more healthy foods because you feel better when you eat them and they keep you feeling satisfied for longer. Plus the lack of processing means they may taste better too.

Eventually, based on your inner and outer wisdoms, you might choose to dramatically change the nutritional balance of what you are eating. Perhaps you'll experiment with being vegetarian, avoiding processed foods, greatly reducing your consumption of dairy, or cutting way back on refined grains. But I invite you to do so without a "food as poison" mind-set.

Unless you or your family members are susceptible to specific food allergies—such as to peanuts or gluten—you might want to be careful not to give into the food phobia fad. Now being labeled *orthorexia*, this phobia is reaching the level of a new eating disorder for some individuals as more and more foods, in any quantity, are rigorously avoided. Being mindful and flexible may seem more challenging than having hard-and-fast unbreakable rules, but in the long term, mindfulness can help you more easily maneuver the complexities of life with a sense of creative exploration and experimentation.

Learning to Love (Or at Least Like) Movement

Though you will not find specific advice in Part Two of the book for how to develop an exercise program, I still encourage you to apply mindfulness to your fitness efforts. Physical activity does a lot more than merely help you firm up or burn extra calories. It reduces risk of developing several diseases, including cardiac disease, type 2 diabetes and some cancers. It also keeps bones and muscles strong, joints more flexible, improves balance, boosts mood, and improves cognitive function and quality of life.[2] It can also boost mood and reduce stress, helping keep emotional eating in check. And it happens to be a wonderful way for you to appreciate your body rather than judge it, as you gradually develop muscle strength and endurance.

You might be surprised to learn, for instance, that it takes a lot less physical activity to benefit your mind and body than you probably think. If you are currently sedentary, it takes only about 75 minutes a week of brisk walking to add nearly 2 years to your life. That's just 10 minutes a day. If you walk twice as much—150 to 299 minutes a week (20 to 40 minutes a day)—you can add more than 3 years. Walk even more—up to 60 minutes daily—and you've added more than 4 years.[3] This is true regardless of your weight level—and the quality of that life will be better throughout.

And movement can include regular daily activities that most of us don't think of as exercise. Consider hotel housekeeping staff. They spend their days lugging heavy equipment, pushing carts, scrubbing, making beds, and walking. Yet when Harvard psychologist Ellen Langer surveyed hotel housekeepers, she found that 67 percent reported that they didn't exercise, though they far exceeded the U.S. Surgeon General's recommendation for daily activity. They thought of what they were doing as only work.[4] Much like those housekeepers, when we walk to the car, run up the stairs, or race down the hallway to a meeting, we don't think, "I'm exercising." But we are.

Use your mindfulness skills to experiment with many different ways to move. With mindfulness, you may find that you enjoy dancing or yoga or any array of options, while you don't enjoy others. You might also discover that using a pedometer helps motivate you to add activity to your day—walking to see that coworker rather than texting or taking the stairs rather than the elevator. Many people in our programs have become excited about adding steps, using the goal we suggest: adding 10 to 20 percent each week, rather than the often recommended 10,000 steps that may feel almost impossible. Your body was made to move, and you will feel better when you do so.

However, if you're not used to exercising, there are two important cautions: build up slowly and avoid the compensation effect! One study found that people who went on a walk and viewed it as exercise then ate a larger portion of dessert at lunch than did those who took the same path, in the same length of time, but viewed it as a nature walk.[5] A number of websites provide lists of exercise/calorie balance, such as NutriStrategy (nutristrategy.com/caloriesburned.htm).

The more mindfulness you cultivate, the easier it will be for you to gain the wisdom needed to design your own fitness routine and to alter that routine as needed. In this way, you'll choose forms of movement that are sustainable, so your success can last.

Breaking Free from the Scale

A final element of outer wisdom is creating a healthy relationship to tracking your weight-loss progress. Many people have an unhealthy relationship with the scale, seeing their weight as an indication of their success or of their self-worth. If they step on the scale and see the number they wanted—perhaps they're down a pound or two—they're happy. If, however, they don't see that number—maybe their weight is the same or higher—they're disappointed. It can color their whole day, and often that disappointment can lead to giving up altogether.

No matter what number you see on the scale, however, it's not an indication of your self-worth. Nor is it a sign of your failure. After all, your metabolism slows as you lose weight, no matter how mindful you are around your eating and movement. You can be mindfully successful, making dozens of positive choices each day for your health, and still not end up seeing a lower number on the scale on a given day.

The number on your scale, however, *is* a way to inform your wisdom. When you work to see that number as information—and nothing more—you can use what you learn to eat even more mindfully and to celebrate your progress. There are several methods that you can use to shift this relationship to a more positive place. I encourage you to pick one (or a combination of them) that is most helpful to *you* for the long term. With a sense of mindfulness, consider which of the following you'd prefer:

Method 1: Experiment with weighing yourself once a week. Once-a-week weighing is more likely to reveal real weight changes, rather than being sensitive to normal 1- to 3-pound daily fluctuations that occur due to water retention and other factors. When you step on the scale once every week or two, you might see changes, but even then a 1- to 2-pound loss can be hidden by daily fluctuations. Being at a plateau for a while also isn't bad; it's time to become comfortable and confident with the changes that you've made. If, on the other hand, your weight is creeping up, rather than saying to yourself, "That's terrible," just consider why that might be, and then ask, "What can I do about this?"

Method 2: Experiment with weighing yourself daily, but only for a week or two. Again, try to be both realistic and kind to yourself. The purpose is to learn what your typical daily fluctuations are and to learn to take those into account. It will also help you become more aware of your judgmental thought patterns, either good or bad, in relation to these daily fluctuations: "Oh, I'm going to have a good day because I'm down 2 pounds." "This is terrible! I'm up a pound, and I tried so hard yesterday." (You know the talk!) Once you become aware of these thought patterns, you're on the road to starting to let go of them and to let go of beating yourself up over tiny, normal, daily fluctuations.

Method 3: Skip the scale (at least regularly) altogether. Use a nonforgiving pair of pants (no elastic waist band, nonstretch material) as your weight-loss yardstick. Maybe they are a pair that once fit, but are now too snug. Or maybe they are a pair that you decide to buy from a thrift shop just to use to gauge your progress. Try them on once a month or so to see if they feel roomier.

No matter what method you use, know that it is impossible to see meaningful results on the scale from day to day. And sometimes, you won't see results on the scale from week to week. That's why I recommend you gauge your progress not with the scale but rather by keeping track of your behavior, thoughts, and feelings. In this approach, you don't focus on the weight. You focus on being able to make more and more of your many daily choices mindfully. In this way, even your mindless eating is now in balance and you continue to feel successful!

Moving On

You've now learned much about the background and core ideas behind mindful eating, and have perhaps tried out a few already. In Part Two, you'll begin to put them into practice. The next chapter provides a self-assessment approach to those dozens of small but important steps in moving from mindless eating to mindful eating and to the big picture of how you're freeing your whole being from that sense of struggle with eating and food. You'll then begin on the path of cultivating mindfulness—and mindful eating.

PART TWO

The Practice of Mindful Eating

CHAPTER SIX

Tools for Getting Started

Part Two of *The Joy of Half a Cookie* follows as much as possible the structure of the 10-week MB-EAT program and related workshops. You'll begin with learning mindfulness meditation and then continue by using mindfulness to cultivate inner and outer wisdom. You'll learn the elements of mindful eating: tuning in to your own hunger experiences, learning to notice when your body and mind are saying "enough," and engaging a broader capacity for mindful awareness so you're less likely to get tripped up by all those old habits left over from many years of struggling.

Using These Practices

Of the following practices, you'll do the first two right away. The first, completing the Keep It Off Checklist for the first time, will help you document your starting point, making it easier for you to track your progress moving toward mindful eating. It will take you just a few minutes to fill out. Then you can put it aside for later.

The second practice, the Circle of Being, will help you rebalance your relationship to eating, weight, and your body, with your relationship to your whole self, as you begin to let go of the sense of struggle that has been there for far too long. Again, this tool helps you document where you are now. You'll complete this again several weeks from now so you can see how much you've changed.

The third practice brings you back to the Keep It Off Checklist, but in a bit of a different way, that you'll use as you progress through the rest of this book.

PRACTICE 1

The Keep It Off Checklist

The Keep It Off Checklist (page 98) is designed to help you stay motivated and feel successful.[1] It takes just a few moments to complete and provides you with a quick look at where you are now as well as some of the specific ways you can create more mindfulness in relation to your eating.

As we've noted, most diets teach very little about changing how you need to eat in a more flexible way in the long run. All of us make many, many small decisions every day about how and what to eat. Shifting these toward a more mindful style of eating is how this program is designed to help you.

Developed for and used in my research, the Keep It Off Checklist will help you notice the dozens of opportunities a day to congratulate and encourage yourself.[2] It encourages you to make *lasting* changes to your relationship to food and lifestyle habits by helping you infuse your effort with realism, self-acceptance, and flexibility. Finally, the checklist is designed to counteract another trap we often set for ourselves when we're trying to make changes: the temptation to go from never to always ("I never leave food on my plate" to "I always leave food on my plate") or from always to never ("I always eat in front of the TV" to "I never eat in front of the TV"). Is that realistic or even necessary? Setting more moderate goals and letting yourself be proud of them is much better.

By using the Keep It Off Checklist, you'll more easily notice and celebrate your growing self-awareness, and you'll make changes that work for *you*.

The list includes many different choices (you can add more) that you might consider in increasing or decreasing long-standing eating habits to create better balance. Instead of focusing primarily on types and amounts of food, it helps you focus more on creating a healthier, more relaxed relationship to eating and with food that you can consider keeping indefinitely, not just until the next "diet" is over. It also includes a way to set goals for yourself that are flexible and realistic, rather than all-or-nothing.

The Practice: Using the Keep It Off Checklist to Track Success

It will only take a few minutes. Follow these steps:

1. **Take a look at the checklist on page 98.** I invite you to photocopy the checklist (so you can come back to it when you like). And to make multiple copies to use again later. Or you can download it and other forms from my website at MB-EAT.com.

2. **Date your sheet, and fill it in now, *before* you've started the practices in the rest of Part Two.** *Note:* If you've already been making changes based on reading through the first half of the book, I welcome you to fill it out based on your older patterns from before you started working with the practices in the book so you can give yourself maximum credit for becoming more mindful!

3. **Rate each item based on how often you engaged in it or experienced it during the past week** (or a recent typical week, if the past week has involved travel or less typical activities). Your possible responses range from "never in the last week" to "several times a day." Avoid the temptation to make yourself look good; that will make it harder to see when you're moving successfully toward more balanced eating! Also, try not to become discouraged as you fill it out. One key purpose of the checklist is to help you stay away from the all-or-nothing thinking that often goes along with changing behavior and losing weight. Going from doing something positive once a week to several times a week might be a great accomplishment. Similarly, going from doing something that's problematic, such as eating because you're upset about something several times a day, to only doing this a few times a week is great and may be what many flexible, Balanced Eaters do.

You can put this original completed Keep It Off Checklist aside for now until you've finished the entire program. And then start a new one for Practice 3 (page 94). In our program, people are usually very surprised when they look back at their original Keep It Off Checklist to see how far they've come, even when they've been keeping track of the smaller changes every few weeks.

Reflections on Practice 1

If you look over your Checklist for some general patterns, you might discover some areas where you realize you are already doing quite well. One woman in a group noted she had tended to get very upset at herself whenever she ate when she was anxious, but then realized that she actually did this only several times per week.

Wait to reassess yourself with the Keep It Off Checklist until you've been working with other practices in Part Two for at least a couple of weeks, and then you can come back to it again every few weeks. Practice 3 will guide you in how to do this. Now it's time to move on to Practice 2.

PRACTICE 2

The Circle of Being

As you embrace mindful eating, your relationship with eating will begin to shift in several ways. One key shift: How you define who you are. When I first meet with new clients, many of them define themselves by their weight and their preoccupation and struggle with food. They see themselves as overeaters, out-of-control, overweight, addicted, or obsessed. Though they certainly may very well be struggling with their eating and spending a lot of time worrying about it, their lives are always richer and fuller than this; they have families, work or school, and other passions. To help them create a better balance between their struggle with food and the other parts of their life, I have them do the following exercise.

The Practice: Bring Balance to the Struggle and to Your Circle of Being

Start the exercise here! Resist the urge to read ahead.

1. **Think about what percentage of your time and energy, in a typical day, you spend on eating, weight, and your body.** Close your eyes. Reflect. How much do you think about, obsess over, and feel badly about your body and your eating? How much time and energy do you spend planning meals, shopping for food, cooking, eating, exercising, and any other tasks involved with eating and weight loss? Some of this energy may be positive: trying out new recipes for your friends or family; experimenting with healthier food choices; exploring sustainability options. For now, just see what percentage number comes to mind.

   It might be 90 percent, 80 percent, 60 percent, 30 percent, even less, or somewhere in between. Just see what number comes to mind for you. Everyone will be different, and there is no right or wrong answer. Don't continue with the practice until you have your number in mind.

2. **On a piece of paper, draw a circle like the one shown on the next page.** The circle represents your total amount of energy, time, thought, and experience during your waking hours (not the full 24-hour day) on a typical day. Each portion of the circle represents about 10 percent of this total time and energy.

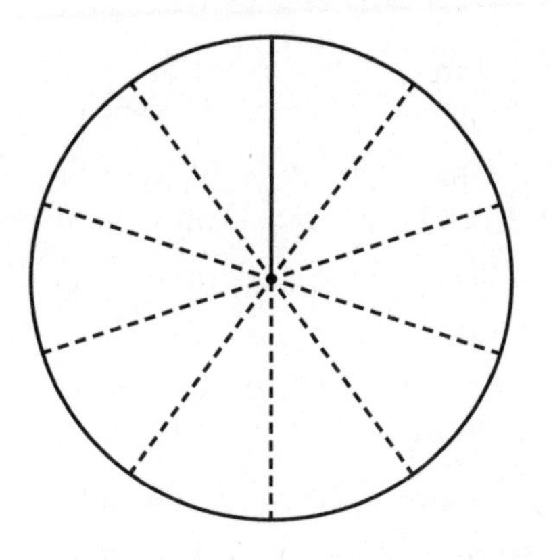

3. **Recall the number that came to mind in step 1** and draw a second dark line that reflects that amount. For example, maybe the number that came to mind in regard to the time and energy you put into eating and weight loss was 50 percent—that's half the circle. Maybe it's 70 percent (seven segments of the circle) or 40 percent (four segments). You can also use half segments if you want to add 5 percent.

4. **Create a list of other important areas of your life** such as family, work, hobbies, volunteering, and spirituality. What other areas of your life, besides eating, food, and your body do you give your time, energy, and attention to during a typical day? Use the side of the paper or a separate sheet.

5. **Reexamine your circle.** Consider that the energy you give to everything else you listed in step 4 must also fit in your circle. You only have one circle of total time and energy. Can all of these other life areas fit into the rest of the circle? For instance, if you designated 75 percent of your circle for energy devoted to concerns about food or weight, does the

rest of your life fit into the remaining 25 percent? Do you really only spend 20 percent of your time at work, for instance? Where does that fit into your circle? What about important hobbies? Your family? Is it possible that you spend a lot less time and energy worrying about food and eating than you think?

Given these other important areas of your life, how might you adjust that first number regarding eating, food, and weight concerns? Does a new number come into your mind right now? There are no exactly right numbers, and they may vary from day to day and week to week. The challenge is to explore what is true for you now, but not to judge it.

6. **Play with your circle over the coming weeks** as you tune in to the time and energy you place on these other parts of your life. As you go through your week, consider how much time you spend on these other important areas of your life. I encourage you to redraw your circle on a new piece of paper several times during a typical week or two until you feel it generally reflects the balance of how you spend your time and energy. In addition to worry or preoccupation with eating and weight, the percentage is intended to also reflect actual activities related to eating, food, appearance, and so on. So be sure to keep that in mind. Most of us do spend meaningful amounts of time cooking, shopping for food, enjoying our meals, and at least a little energy on our appearance. Some of us work in an occupation that entails giving substantial amounts of time to these areas. That's, of course, fine. We're talking about recognizing what this balance actually is and whether you wish to adjust it.

7. **Consider what you would like your circle to look like.** Are you putting time and energy into what matters most to you? Are you putting too much time and energy into activities that you don't value very highly? Consider what proportions might best reflect your real values to create a healthy and happy balance, as you decrease the struggle with eating and weight. Consider what might be an appropriate amount of time to give to these issues, including time spent engaging in meal preparation, eating more mindfully, exercising, and taking care of your body.

Reflections on Practice 2

Again, there are no exactly right numbers for the Circle of Being. Everyone is different. The point is to acknowledge the role food and eating play in your life, relative to other things you value, and then to decide how large of a role you want these to play. Notice that the worry and preoccupation with your weight and eating takes up time and energy that might more pleasantly and even joyfully be spent elsewhere. We all have moments of a wandering mind when we're not focused, busy, or being mindful. That's fine and normal and can include pleasant meandering daydreams, creative space, and many, many other things. But if your wandering mind always clicks onto worries about your body, appearance, or weight, then you are taking away energy from other possibilities. Being mindful and more self-accepting may open up surprising space.

When I did this practice with Susan, she said that 85 percent was the number that came into her mind. She wanted to lose about 30 pounds and had tried multiple diets on which she would lose about 15 pounds and then regain the weight. She wanted to try something different, partly because she was concerned that her children, including her teenage daughter, were picking up bad habits from her and because she was afraid she was being passed over at work for a promotion because of how heavy she was. Clearly, she had many other aspects of her life that were important to her. In doing this exercise, she was able to immediately reconsider her first number of 85 percent and drop it down to about 65 percent. As her capacity for mindfulness increased and her increased sense of confidence around eating grew, she also caught herself when she began obsessing needlessly over her weight and eating, and began to let go of such worries when they arose. Over the course of the program, she realized she could bring all her issues with eating, food, and weight into better balance with the rest of her life and yet be even more effective with making wiser decisions regarding how she and her family were eating. At the end of the program, she had dropped that initial 85 percent down to 30 percent.

PRACTICE 3

Incorporating Mindful Changes into Your Life

Practice 3 picks up where Practice 1 ends and involves filling out the Keep It Off Checklist again and again over time to see how many mindful changes you've incorporated into your life. Return to this practice at regular intervals, perhaps as often as once every week or two.

1. **Fill out a fresh copy of the Keep It Off Checklist.** Use a single copy of the checklist, adding to it each week, or use a blank copy of the checklist each time.

2. **As you fill out the checklist, reflect on the previous week.** Compare your results to your original responses. If you see any changes, take note of those first. Well done!

3. **In each section, consider adding more items** if you wish, to identify other meaningful patterns you've become aware of that aren't on the original Keep It Off Checklist.

4. **Pick three to four items to target for making small changes during the next week.** I suggest choosing ones that you feel particularly drawn to and that are related to what you've been reading and practicing.

5. **Keep in mind that your goal on these items is to move only one or two steps,** not from "never" to "always" or vice versa. Instead, you might move from "several times a day" to "once a day" or from "never" to "at least once a week."

6. **Reflect again on the changes you've targeted to make sure they are realistic.** On a scale of 1 to 10, with 1 being "not likely" and 10 being "definitely likely," how likely is it that you could make each change permanent (even if it's just going from "never" to "once per week")? If your answer to any of them is "not likely," you might consider choosing a different goal and coming back to the more challenging one later, when you have more experience. But if it's in between, that's fine.

7. **Plan how you'll work with each goal.** Think about when and how you might make changes. Which days? Which meals? Which foods?

8. **Consider the value of particular changes for the long run.** How will they make your life better? How will they alter your relationship with food? How will they bring you

more pleasure, joy, and inner peace? How will they reduce the struggle and give you a sense of freedom?

9. **Approach this journey with an attitude of curiosity and exploration.** It may be that something you thought would be difficult is now a lot easier than you expected, given your new mindfulness skills. Or perhaps you'll discover that a change you planned is proving to be difficult and perhaps even one that you may need to reconsider doing.

Reflections on Practice 3

Stay with your three or four goals for at least a week or so, before moving on to another set, or increasing or decreasing your frequency. Find small steps that are realistic in both the short term and the long term. In this way, you'll gradually shift long-standing patterns, and you'll feel great about making those changes!

Keep in mind that the road to lasting change involves a process of experimentation and exploration, self-awareness and self-acceptance. Something you thought would be hard may turn out to be easy, at least if you're not going from always to never. And conversely, you might be surprised how difficult something is that you thought, at first, might be easy. If so, are there ways you can adapt your goal to make it more realistic?

Think about your choices both in the short term—during this coming week—and in the long term—changes you'd like to slowly make, perhaps over a year's time, which you can adapt to your life. For instance, a longer-term goal might be savoring every bite while you are in the middle of a party. A shorter-term goal might be to fully savor the first few bites of a meal that you are eating alone without any distractions.

Come back to the Keep It Off Checklist over and over again as you navigate the rest of the book. Your answers will change over time, and you can use them to see just how much more mindful you are becoming compared to when you started. Every now and then you might compare where you are now with your very first record. When we do that in our program after about two months, most people are quite startled and pleased to see how far they've come in letting go of the struggle and becoming more mindful.

It might take a month, give or take, before new changes feel like habits. Continue to set goals at whatever pace seems to work best for you. Eventually, you'll find that you are practicing more and more of the wisdom skills of mindful eating consistently.

Moving On

No matter how you rate yourself on your evolving relationship to your eating and food, know this: You can experiment and you can move forward with new mindful skills. Just as learning a new language, a musical instrument, or a new task at work requires study and practice, so does learning this new way of relating to food and eating. Embark on this journey with a sense of curiosity. Remain flexible, see each practice as an experiment, and celebrate every success along the way. Continually reinforce yourself by rejoicing over what you are already doing well ("Wow, I really savored the first bite of this meal!" "Wow, I just left food on my plate and didn't feel guilty about it!" "Wow, I stopped eating before I felt at all uncomfortable!") as well as by noticing opportunities to improve even more. You have dozens if not hundreds of opportunities a day to congratulate and encourage yourself. Also notice how letting go of the struggle may be freeing up energy for other valuable parts of your life: your family, your work, and whatever else you hold dear.

The Keep It Off Checklist

Mindful Eating Skills to Do More Often
1. I noticed when I was physically hungry.
2. I stopped eating when I began to feel comfortably full.
3. I stopped eating when I noticed I wasn't tasting the food as much.
4. I ate slowly and mindfully, fully experiencing each bite.
5. I stopped eating something because it tasted too sweet, too fatty, or too salty.
6. I decided not to eat a tempting food, thinking, "I can always have it some other time."
7. I ate something I like very much without eating too much of it.
8. I let myself really enjoy and savor all the flavor and textures in a meal.
9. I ate moderately at a social gathering.
10. I added more healthy foods to my regular diet.
11. I reduced the amount of unhealthy foods in my regular diet.
12. I decided not to take a second helping because I was already satisfied.
13. I figured out the number of calories of a food before I ate it.
14. I ate a smaller portion of something I wanted in order to reduce overall calories.

1 = never in the last week	2 = at least once in the last week	3 = several times in the last week	4 = once a day	5 = several times a day	N/A = not applicable

The Keep It Off Checklist *(continued)*

Mindless or Restrictive Behaviors and Thoughts to Do Less Often
I overate after feeling upset about something.
I ate something fattening and then kept on eating because "I'd already blown it."
I ate because I was putting off doing something else.
I finished everything on my plate (or all of a snack) without checking whether I'd already had enough.
I ate just because I was bored.
I ate most of a snack or meal mindlessly.
I avoided checking calories of something because it made me too anxious.
I spent too much time worrying about my weight, my appearance, and my eating.
I weighed myself out of worry/concern.
Other Mindful Lifestyle Behaviors
I practiced meditation for at least 10 minutes.
I practiced meditation for at least 20 minutes.
I weighed myself, just to inform my wisdom, rather than to police myself.
I purposefully built more activity into my day.
While exercising (or just being more active), I appreciated my body for what it can do instead of what it can't do.

1 = never in the last week	2 = at least once in the last week	3 = several times in the last week	4 = once a day	5 = several times a day	N/A = not applicable

Using the Rest of the Chapters

In general, I suggest that you read and make use of the exercises in the chapters that follow in the order they are presented, trying most of the practices as you get to them, saving some more advanced variations for later, and then revisiting core practices over and over again as they become easier and easier. Each chapter will provide more guidance in how to best do this. It doesn't have to take you 10 weeks (the length of the full MB-EAT program) to go through everything. On the other hand, 10 weeks isn't very long to shift patterns that you may have been living with for years.

CHAPTER SEVEN

Mindfulness 101

It's time to get started with three practices that will serve as the foundation for the rest of your journey: mindfulness meditation, mini-meditations, and your first mindful eating experience. They provide the foundation of mindfulness, which is a special quality of awareness and attention.

This important trio of mindfulness practices will help you:

Bring your attention to the present. Our brains process thousands of bits of information every minute. Whatever is most salient or most important comes into conscious awareness, yet much of how we respond is automatic. As you learn to focus on your breathing, you'll become more aware of your mind wandering to different thoughts, feelings, and memories, and you'll learn how to better direct your attention toward where you wish it to go, rather than feeling as if it were an automatic process. This mind wandering is a natural and normal process, but you'll find more and more that you are able to, quietly and without judgment, direct your mind rather than having your mind direct you.

No matter how weak or how strong your powers of attention are, you can improve, and you can become more mindfully aware. You may find, as some people do, that your mind quiets down almost immediately, with that intrusive internal chattering showing up only occasionally. Or you may find that you're far more aware of how much chattering there is going on in your mind. That's fine also—that's the first step of helping it gradually quiet down. Over time, that seemingly incessant chattering will continue to soften and slow. Yet even highly experienced meditators will have days when their mind is racing, perhaps because of unusually high stress or an impending life decision. Some people in our workshops struggle a little more with this because they have attention deficit disorder. It does take them longer to find that place of quiet focus, but when they do, they are amazed at the value it brings to their entire life.

Tune in to your experiences, without judgment. Just as lifting weights over and over again strengthens your muscles so you feel stronger and more confident whatever your activity, focusing on your breath, thoughts, and feelings will strengthen your ability to tune in and become more aware of your inner experience, whatever the situation. The more focused your attention, the better your ability to place it wherever you want—on your sensations of hunger and fullness, the awareness of tasting your food, and the thoughts that bring you peace of mind—rather than on feelings of guilt and anxiety.

Doing this without judgment means to first notice and then let go of all those critical inner voices that are making evaluative judgments about the thoughts and feelings that arise. Judgment itself is part of human nature, but it also takes us away from our immediate experience. This applies to our experiences of eating and food and much of the rest of our life.

Food is a gift you offer to your body. Food nourishes your cells with the raw materials they need for health. It also nourishes your senses. We live in a world with more food choices than has ever been possible. You can either engage this mindlessly and anxiously or be respectful and even joyful about these possibilities. When you are not only mindful of your choices and your experience but also appreciative of them, you'll transform every single meal, without a sense of struggle and without overeating.

Tap into your inner wisdom. As you learn how to rest your mind on the breath and then on the practice of eating, you will become more and more aware of your desires, hunger, emotions, and other eating triggers, and you can make wiser decisions about what and what not to eat. If you recall the image of moving from the chattering mind to the thinking mind to the wise mind, you can envision that this process will help you in handling all types of decisions and choices in relation to food in a more powerful, yet satisfying way. You'll learn how to *respond* rather than *react.*

Rather than immediately seeing a food and thinking, "I want this. I shouldn't. I can't. I'll overeat it," you'll be able to rest your awareness on the food for a few moments to better appreciate your possibilities: "Eat nothing because I'm really not hungry." "Save for later." "Eat some right now but make sure to taste every bite." "Eat something else." And so on. As you pause for a few moments, you may be surprised as the wiser alternatives come into awareness, often with one seeming just right for that moment. But all this takes practice, and that practice starts with mindful awareness of the breath.

The Benefits of Focusing on the Breath

Once you learn how to become aware of and focused on your breathing, you'll be developing the skills to become more aware of and focused on anything, including your sensations of hunger, fullness, desire, thoughts, and emotions. As a tool to hone your mindful awareness, attending to the breath is powerful because:

- **Your breath is always there.** Thus you can meditate on the breath at any time of the day or night, and you need no special equipment. Just close your eyes and tune in. Once you become used to meditating on the breath, you don't even need to close your eyes. You can do it in front of other people, and no one will know what you are doing.
- **The breath is one of the fundamental links between your mind and your body.** When we take short, rapid breaths, we're often anxious, angry, or afraid because such breathing might help us react more quickly in an emergency. Deeper, slower breaths go with being relaxed and calm. When we purposefully shift from fast, shallow breathing, to slower, deeper breathing, we're giving our brain the message that we don't need to breathe faster, and we automatically relax. So by slowing down and taking deeper breaths, you can shift your mood to one of awareness rather than reaction.
- **The breath is rhythmical.** Many contemplative practices rely on rhythm, including some prayers, chanting, Sufi dancing, and drumming. By moving to or focusing on a rhythm—in this case, the breath—we interrupt our preoccupied, obsessive mind and move to a more neutral or relaxed state.

- **Breathing is linked to wisdom.** The Latin root for the word *breathe* is "spiro," related in English to *spirit* and *inspiration.* In this way, our language links breathing with wisdom and spirituality. This is true of other languages. For instance, in Chinese and Japanese, *qi*, or *chi*, means "breath" as well as "life force" or "life energy."

Using These Practices

If you wish, you can do all of the following practices in one session or you can spread them out over a few days, but I suggest you do them in the order they are presented. Then consider giving yourself a week of simply experiencing the value of these practices before moving on to those in the next chapter.

PRACTICE 1

Breathe Mindfully

If you've never meditated before, the very thought of it may feel intimidating. But the process is very simple: choosing a time and place of quiet sitting so you won't be likely to fall asleep; attending to the quality and rhythm of your breath; and practicing noticing, without judgment, the thoughts, feelings, and experiences that arise. Then stopping at the end of the time that you've allotted. Plan to meditate for 10 to 20 minutes (see page 109 for more instructions or use either the 10- or the 20-minute audio guide available at www.mb-eat.com).

Choose a quiet time and area to do your meditation practice. Morning is the best time, as it is a way to set your mind for the day, and you are far less likely to feel drowsy, which can be an issue later in the evening. But other times of day may work well for you. If you're not using the audio guide, set a timer to track how long you meditate. (Depending how loud it is, you might put the timer in a nearby room, so you're not too startled when it goes off.) If feasible, mute the ringer on your phone. If you are at home but not alone, you might sit where you won't be distracted by family members and ask them to provide you with private time. If you have young children (or even a forgetful spouse), you might find it helpful to set a timer for them for a few minutes longer than you plan to practice.

The rest is as simple as sitting comfortably, closing your eyes, and following your breath with your mind.

Advice on Sitting Comfortably

You might have seen pictures of people meditating in the lotus posture, crossed legged with each foot on the opposite thigh. If your knees hurt just thinking about it, relax. You don't need to look like a Zen master or yogi in order to meditate.

Your goal is to find a position that is comfortable enough that you aren't distracted by pain or discomfort in your feet, knees, or back. At the same time, you don't want to be so comfortable that your mind zones out or you fall asleep.

For most people, that means you'll be sitting on either a chair or the floor on a cushion (or two).

If you choose a chair:

- Pick an upright but comfortable chair with a firm back. It's hard to stay alert when your eyes are closed, everything is quiet, and you are in a soft, plush chair or sofa that swallows you up.
- Place your feet flat on the floor. If your legs are short, place them on a cushion so they are firmly supported. Crossing your legs will quickly come to feel imbalanced.

If you choose the floor:

- Prop up your bottom with a 3- to 6-inch-thick cushion or pillow, so your hips are higher than your feet. This will help alleviate tension in your back.
- If your flooring is wood, tile, or some other hard surface, place a yoga mat or blanket under the cushion. This will protect your feet, ankles and legs from becoming too uncomfortable.

Whether you are seated on the floor or on a chair, sit tall, with the crown of your head toward the ceiling. Lower your chin, tucking it slightly inward. This will lengthen and relax the back of your neck, resulting in a more comfortable practice. To tell if your spine is balanced, rock forward and back until you find a position that feels just right—not too far forward and not too far back. If you're on a chair, sit a few inches away from the back of it to start strengthening your back muscles. If, after a while, you feel uncomfortable—maybe your feet fall asleep, you have a nagging ache in your back, or even find that you have an itch begging you to scratch it, go ahead and, with intention, move enough to become more comfortable. Just keep your mind on what you are doing. If you need to relax against the back of the chair for a few minutes, then do so, mindfully, and then try again in a few minutes to sit more upright without using the back support. In this way, you'll gradually strengthen those back muscles.

The Practice: Breathing Mindfully

Once you are ready, follow this sequence:

1. **Begin to breathe from your abdomen.** Start with three or four deeper breaths, letting your shoulders relax, your stom-

ach relax. Your stomach should expand as you breathe in and then relax and sink down as you breathe out. To check if you are breathing correctly, place your right hand on your stomach and your left on your chest. If your right hand rises and falls with the breath as your left hand stays still, you are breathing from the right area of your body. If you are a usually a chest breather, this new way of breathing might feel uncomfortable at first. Don't worry. It will eventually become second nature. This type of breathing also sends a signal back to your brain that you are really are relaxed.

2. **Let your breath slow down to a usual rhythm and pace.** There's no need to exaggerate your breathing or to continue to take deeper or fuller breaths than usual.

3. **Follow your breath.** As you inhale, notice the air at the tip of your nose cool as it flows in. Continue by observing it as moves down the back of your throat, into your abdomen and then back out again, now warmer at the tip of your nostrils as it flows out.

4. **When your attention wanders, simply bring it back to your breath.** It is natural and normal for your awareness to shift off your breath to other experiences, such as thoughts, feelings, or sounds. Indeed, it is an important part of the practice to simply notice that this has happened, without judgment, and then gently return your awareness back to the breath.

   Notice every new sensation: the feeling of air at the tip of your nose, the expansion in your torso, the rising of your belly.

5. **Explore and experiment!** If there is a particular place where the feel of your breath is clearer—the tip of your nose, the back of your throat, the rise and fall of your stomach—then choose that as the primary focus for your awareness. Or choose to follow the entire course of your breath.

Breath Awareness Mindfulness Meditation Practice

If you prefer to be guided through this breathing meditation, you can download this and other meditations from www.mb-eat.com. You might begin with the 10-minute practice, with detailed instructions, for the first week. Then move to the 10-minute practice with brief instructions for another week. Then do the 20-minute practice. You may wish to extend the practice to 30 or even 40 minutes, a more traditional length, as some people prefer. After a few weeks you may find that you don't really need to listen to the audio guide at all in order to practice, and you might simply use a timer.

Reflections on Practice 1

As with learning any new skill, daily practice will help you create a routine. Just as you never forget to shower or brush your teeth, you'll find you can work it more and more easily into your daily routine. In the beginning, however, if you miss a day or two, don't be hard on yourself. Just start again.

As you practice, consider setting short-term, realistic goals for yourself. Rather than expecting yourself to stay focused on your breath for an entire 10- or 20-minute session (not possible!), your first goal might be to follow your breathing for 20 breaths, without losing count. Then for 30 breaths, 50, and on up to 100. You might use counting once a week or so to see how you are doing with this. If you tend to be a competitive person, be gentle with yourself. In my experience, it takes most people around a year or more to stay aware for 100 breaths. Even when you are counting, this doesn't mean that your mind is only on your breath for the entire time. You will still notice thoughts, sounds, or feelings; you just don't become so absorbed in them that you lose track of the count. As long as you keep practicing, you'll develop a higher and higher level of sustained awareness.

My workshop participants often raise the following questions about this practice:

How will I ever find 10 spare minutes to meditate?

If you are very busy, see your mindfulness practice as a wonderful gift of space and time, rather than a burden. You probably spend 10 to 20 minutes a day involved in many different pursuits that offer you much less benefit. You might spend 10 minutes a day reading a newspaper or magazine, watching television, surfing the Web, or chatting on the phone. Unlike many pursuits, every moment you spend cultivating mindful awareness is time well spent. You couldn't be spending your time any more wisely. So whenever you feel tempted to make the excuse "I'm too busy," tell yourself, "That means I need to meditate."

When I do belly breathing, I feel light headed. Is this normal?

It's normal, but not ideal. You may be breathing too quickly and too deeply, and not fully exhaling. So slow down your breathing, perhaps counting slowly to four on each inhalation, pausing slightly, and on each exhalation counting again to four, or even five or six, making sure to fully exhale before bringing in another breath.

When I meditate, why do I sometimes feel like I'm almost floating?

We know where our bodies are because of constant feedback from all our joints and muscles. Without that feedback, even if subtle, we may lose that sense of body presence. So when this happens, it means you've become able to sit very still!

What should I do if I can't stop thinking?

Even if at first your mind becomes quiet and relaxed, you will probably get distracted. You might notice sounds around you. Your right foot might start itching. Your thoughts might chatter along (Am I doing this right? I wonder what's on TV tonight? Oh, did I put the laundry in the dryer?). Memories might surface. Your wandering mind might go to a mental to-do list or become involved in daydreams. Noticing and then letting go of judgment thoughts ("I shouldn't have done that!" "I should have done that!" "I hate that noise!" "Why can't I stop thinking about that itch?") can be harder. Again the first step is simply to notice them ("Ah, a judgment thought." "Ah, an itch." "Ah, restlessness."), and then let go of the urge to react. It will become easier.

Every time you realize you've gotten lost in a line of thought (as we often do during our usual thinking day), just observe that it happened and then gently, over and over, bring yourself back to your breath.

Let me share an image. Imagine yourself sitting on the bank of a lovely stream. Watching the ripples of the water flow by is like watching the rise and fall of your breath. But then you notice a leaf in the water. Our usual thought process might be this: "Ah, pretty red leaf! A maple leaf! Oh, I forgot to call the lawn people to pick up the leaves. They might be busy—hmmm, I'll see if the neighbor's son can do the raking. Haven't really talked to them since August. I wonder how their trip to Mexico was? Maybe we'll go next year." And so on and so on. With mindful awareness, you also notice the leaf, and that it's red, and perhaps recognize that it's a maple leaf, and that it's pretty. But then you return back to watching the stream, rather than meandering through the usual free associations that we often have. As you practice, you'll notice sooner and sooner when your mind has started wandering, and you can then gently bring it back to your breath—over and over and over.

But if this is really hard to do (and it will be at the beginning), and your thoughts become overly persistent, try one of the following for a few minutes until the chattering or wandering mind quiets and you can return to just the breath:

- **Count with each breath** to 10 a few times. This will help shift your chattering mind onto something that is concrete, quieting down those thoughts.
- **For a few moments, focus on a simple mantra**, such as *Om*, *peace*, or *one*, or some other word. Just don't use the name of a person you know—too many associations! Repeat this mantra silently on the rhythm of your breath.
- **Label your thoughts.** Succinctly describe your thoughts, with a word such as *planning*, *worrying*, or *emotion*. For example, let's say you are meditating and you think, "I have to go take care of this one thing . . ." you could label it *restless*.

Labeling provides a little distance between your thoughts and your response to those thoughts.

Every time you bring yourself back to your breath, you are training your mind. Being aware of your chattering or thinking mind is a huge accomplishment, creating a path into the wise mind. So feel good rather than discouraged every time you catch your wandering mind. Eventually, over time, your mind will wander less and less, and your ability to focus in the moment will improve.

When I try to meditate, even for a few minutes, I find I have thoughts and memories come up that are disturbing, and it feels very uncomfortable. What should I do?

Sometimes these distressing memories or thoughts will simply pass, giving you a sense of awareness, but sometimes they may signal something that needs more wakeful attention. They may even suggest the need to address these issues with a professional therapist, as they can be related to previous trauma in your life or other issues that aren't yet resolved. You may also be able to manage or interrupt these experiences by briefly opening your eyes, by observing these thoughts or images as if on a movie screen, or by using only mini-meditations (see Practice 2 on page 118) to help cultivate becoming more aware of your experiences.

What can I do if I am surrounded by too many distractions?

Perhaps your neighbor is mowing the lawn, there is loud traffic, or your dog keeps bothering you. Rather than berating yourself for noticing what's going on around you, congratulate yourself for being aware. During her first week of meditation, one woman couldn't find any solution for her rambunctious dog. As she sat, the dog restlessly paced, nosed her, and whined. I suggested she try a "What Is My Dog Doing Now?" meditation. Rather than react to her dog by getting up to placate him or being irritated, I suggested she stay seated and follow the dog with her mind. "That's where your awareness is going anyway. So allow yourself to be fully aware of what your dog is doing," I said. During a subsequent session, she said, "It's amazing! He's not driving me crazy anymore. My dog has quieted down. He just sits next to me when I meditate." Another individual realized she could simply observe the train whistle she sometimes heard from her house—rather than observing her irritation at it. She then was surprised that she noticed it less and less.

My friend attends a local meditation group, and that's all the practice she does. Is it okay if I go to that, rather than meditating at home?

You might plan to do both. The group can provide valuable support, but more frequent practicing deepens your skills. Research is showing that regular practice of 20 minutes or so improves your ability to be more mindful and use the mindful eating skills more effectively. What if you were learning to play a musical instrument? Just going to lessons once a week would not be enough. You have to practice to really learn to play.

I've learned to do meditation by using a mantra. Why can't I keep doing that for my meditation practice? It's really relaxing and calming.

Mantra meditation can have tremendous value because your mind has something more concrete (a word or sound) to focus on than the breath. But it may not be as useful in cultivating your ability to simply observe other experiences as they arise, which is the nature and purpose of mindfulness practice. Finally, if you can train yourself to focus on something as neutral as the breath, you will be able to bring focus to almost anything, including thoughts, feelings, or other experiences as they arise—both while you are meditating and during your usual day. Attending to the breath creates more space to gently shift to something else quickly, such as your experience of eating. Attending to a mantra may block out those other experiences, which is sometimes helpful and sometimes not.

You Know You Are Meditating When . . .

You realize that you can't fully quiet your mind. Meditation is not about making your mind go blank. It's about observing, without reacting or following the thoughts or urges, like the maple leaf example given on page 114. If you notice your thoughts, that means you are aware and that you are doing something right and not something wrong. Some thoughts or feelings may be very important ones to be aware of. Others may just be flying through. Just acknowledge them ("Oh, I'm thinking about my 'to-do' list") and return to the breath. You may be surprised at how quickly such thoughts lose their power.

It feels challenging. You are training your mind, again not unlike training a muscle. If you started a new exercise program, you wouldn't think, "I'm breathing hard. I must be doing something wrong." You'd know that with more practice, your breath will quiet down. So will your racing thoughts, sense of impatience, or sense of restlessness, as you continue to meditate.

You are not zoning out. While some meditation traditions lead you into a deeply relaxed, trance-like state, that is not the intention of what we are doing here. Mindfulness is about falling awake, not falling asleep. It's the opposite of a trance. Mindfulness builds your ability to be fully present during every moment of your day, especially during eating. At the same time, as you practice, you may find yourself moving into a state of deep relaxation and inner peacefulness, for a few minutes or eventually for most of your practice, and it can be very soothing. As you continue, you may find you can engage that sense of peacefulness even when faced with difficult challenges in the middle of your active day.

PRACTICE 2

Mini-Meditations

While longer meditation practices train you to bring a quality of focused awareness into every aspect of your everyday life, mini-meditations will help you during everyday situations, and especially before and during meals.

These meditations are exactly as they sound: short mindfulness moments. The mini-meditations might last as long as minute or two or for only a few seconds as you gently bring your racing mind onto something that you wish to observe—like a thought, a feeling, how physically hungry you are, or the delicious taste of a few bites of your favorite dessert.

You can close your eyes if you'd like, but eventually your goal is to be able to do these short meditations anywhere, eyes open or closed, seated or standing. With your eyes open, no one will know you are practicing. Yet, even in the middle of a busy restaurant or an important business lunch, you'll be able to become more aware of your hunger, the food that may be in front of you, and your thoughts and feelings about what you plan to eat. You'll be able to bring your attention to where you want it to be, rather than have it always go to wherever it gets pulled.

The Practice: Doing Mini-Meditations

When you are ready to try mini-meditations:

1. **Initially, take several deep breaths.** Remember to allow the air to flow all the way into your abdomen. If you notice tension in your body, imagine that you are breathing through these areas as you exhale, allowing your breath to relax your muscles. Then let your breathing slow down to a usual pace. You may find you don't always need the deeper breaths to do a mini-meditation, but at first they can be very helpful to signal your mind and body what your intention is.

2. **Become aware of your mind and direct your attention as you wish.** You might want to attend to feelings, sensations in your body, or thoughts, such as the one that's just arisen that you really want some ice cream! Is that because you're really hungry? Or because you just saw an ad for your favorite brand? Or perhaps both?

3. **Don't judge what you discover.** Just become aware of it all. You are cultivating your ability to take a few minutes to observe your experience and then to *choose* how to respond, rather than reacting automatically.

Reflections on Practice 2

Do mini-meditations as often as you want during the day, but especially before and during meals. As you become more familiar with this process, you'll be able to do mini-meditations quickly, in any situation, without closing your eyes. This allows you to bring awareness into any activity. I probably do about 100 a day! Practice whenever you have small snippets of free time: in your car at a light, while standing in line at the grocery store, when waiting for that friend who is running late. With your eyes open, mentally shift your awareness to your thoughts, feelings, and sensations, asking yourself questions like, How do I feel? What is going through my mind? What's happening here? Over time you will naturally become more aware of your thoughts, emotions, and behaviors, which, until recently, were automatic and often took place without your attention. For example, doing a mini-meditation when you're stopped in traffic might first lead you to be aware of how irritated you are becoming, noticing the physical tension and thoughts related to that, including negative judgments (Why can't they time the lights better?). But then you might realize that, if you slow your breath, you can let go of some of this reaction. Eventually you might be able to open your awareness and wisdom to a more positive use of those few minutes!

What happens if you just keep forgetting to do mini-meditations? This is a common concern. One solution is to decide to practice one before every meal or before a particular meal each day, perhaps one you generally eat by yourself. Another way to remind yourself is to place some little stickers (like smiley faces, flowers, or whatever feels appealing) in strategic places, especially in your kitchen, to remind yourself to check in. Maybe you put one on the cabinet where you store your most tempting snack foods. Or perhaps even on the bag or box of a certain food that you tend to consume mindlessly. This isn't about policing yourself. These stickers are merely reminders for you to check in.

Your sticker can even be imaginary. Jane, one of my workshop participants, knew that she tended to snack at work whenever she was under a lot of pressure. At first she put a sticker by her computer screen, but she got so used to it there that she didn't notice the sticker anymore. She then put one on her office doorframe, so she could see it whenever she headed out to meetings. She also realized that much of her stress was related to her boss. So I suggested to her that she imagine a sticker on her boss's forehead whenever she saw him! Since her boss was often the trigger that led to her stress eating, the visualization worked wonderfully.

PRACTICE 3

Mindfully Eating Four Raisins

As soon as you are comfortable with mini-meditations, you can start to cultivate your ability to eat mindfully. This can be on the same day you first start practicing the mini-meditations, or give yourself a little more time to work with them. I borrowed the practice of mindfully eating raisins from Jon Kabat-Zinn's hallmark MBSR program but adapted it to push the envelope of awareness a little further. You can consume any food mindfully, but let's start with raisins. They're a simple food, and consider how we usually eat them—mindlessly, by the handful.

It doesn't matter whether raisins are one of your favorite foods, whether you are neutral about them, or whether you don't even like them much (or you can use dried cranberries instead). You'll still benefit from this practice as it is about experiencing raisins in a new way. And even if you've done this practice before, this version is about experiencing them yet again in a new way.

Before trying the practice, make sure you have some decent quality raisins. Set aside at least 15 minutes, without interruption, to fully experience this mindful eating practice.

You can find a guided practice for mindfully eating raisins at www.mb-eat.com, or you may lead yourself through it following the text. Using the online meditation at least once will be helpful, however, because the pace and experience will carry over to all the other practices in this book. Regardless, you might read through the instructions in the book because they complement each other. But wait until **after** doing the practice to read the Reflections section on page 124.

The Practice: Eating Mindfully

Place four raisins on a napkin or plate in front of you. Then close your eyes, focusing and calming yourself with a few deep breaths, as in doing a mini-meditation.

1. **Staying in this focused, relaxed state, open your eyes and choose one raisin,** looking at it with fresh eyes, as if you've never before eaten or even seen a raisin. What do you notice? What does this raisin look like? Notice its size and its texture. Now, closing your eyes, bring it up to your nose. How does it smell? How does it feel when you gently rub it along the outsides of your lips?

2. **Keeping your eyes closed, place the raisin in your mouth for a few moments** (perhaps to the count of five), *without* chewing it. Just gently hold it with your tongue, moving it around, and noticing how it feels and tastes.

3. **Begin slowly chewing it, experiencing every bit of its taste.** How does the taste change as you bite into the raisin?

Does it change as you continue to chew? What part of your mouth is chewing the raisin in each moment? When do you feel the impulse to swallow? What does it feel like? Continue chewing the raisin, until you've extracted every bit of pleasure from it. Once you swallow the raisin, what do you continue to sense and taste?

4. **Do the same with the second raisin, and then the third,** experiencing each with all of your senses. Take your time, making sure you don't rush yourself. With these raisins, notice how they are similar—and different—from each other, in regard to texture, smell, taste. Any surprises? Be aware that you are taking the food energy of these three little raisins into your body.

5. **Notice your thoughts and feelings throughout.** Are they judging the raisin or judging your reaction to the raisin? ("Wow, this is harder than I expected. This seems a little silly. Hmm, I wish I'd bought a fresh box."). With the third raisin, you might consider what you know about raisins—where are they grown? How are they harvested? Packaged? How do they make their way from there to you? Who are all the people that make that possible, from the farmer to the store cashier? As you do this, continue chewing them mindfully until you've extracted the maximum taste and pleasure from them, and then, mindfully, decide to swallow, bringing this tiny bit of food energy down into your body.

6. **When you get to the fourth raisin, pause and consider: Do you really want it?** Make a decision of whether to

pick up the raisin and eat it, or whether to leave it. Try not to make this decision ahead of time, but consider it in the moment only once you have finished the other three. Now if you decide to go ahead, eat this fourth raisin with as much mindful appreciation as you did with the first three, noticing taste, texture, and your thoughts and feelings.

7. **Regardless of whether you ate the fourth raisin, reflect on how you make this decision**. What was the decision process? Your thoughts, concerns, worries?

8. **End with bringing your awareness back to the breath.** Take two or three deeper breaths. Bring your awareness back to your body and open your eyes.

Reflections on Practice 3

Remember, wait until after you've done the practice to read this section.

Consider how this experience was similar to and different from your usual way of eating raisins or other similar foods. How do you usually eat raisins? And did the raisins taste different from what you expected? If so, how? Any other surprises? What kinds of thoughts ran through your mind during the exercise? What emotions?

Did you conclude, as the participants in my workshops often do, that the taste of the third raisin wasn't quite as good as the first? When I give participants the choice of whether to eat the fourth raisin or not, some find that they really don't have a strong urge to do so. Still their thoughts are battling: "Should I eat another one? Shouldn't I? Do I want more? Should I eat more? I don't want to, but the raisin is there. Should I really just leave it? But I was told never to leave food!" When they see that this internal battle is merely a creation of their ideas about leaving food and self-restraint, it's revealing, and it helps them tap into their own wise mind. So explore what happens for you in this regard, perhaps considering whether you ever have such thoughts when deciding to eat another bite of other types of food.

Moving On

You are now developing the foundation for beginning to eat mindfully. I encourage you to practice what you've just learned for a few days to a week before moving on to the next chapter. Continue to practice sitting meditation and the mini-meditations, as they are the priceless way of bringing this capacity into all parts of your life. As for mindfully eating small bites of food, we'll be asking you to bring that practice into your everyday life little by little, day by day, by mindfully experiencing more and more foods this way over time. Those few minutes you spent with the raisins will now help you bring a new quality to other experiences of eating as you move through the next chapters. I think you'll start to enjoy eating in a way you may never have before.

In the next three chapters, we are going to first provide you with experience with the core inner wisdom practices of awareness of hunger, taste, and fullness. Then you'll be ready for the outer wisdom practices, including the 500-Calorie Challenge, in Chapter 11. As you move ahead, you'll start to link your inner wisdom and outer wisdom skills together in a powerful way.

CHAPTER EIGHT

Feeling True Hunger

Now that you've spent a week or more exploring mindfulness meditation and mindful eating, it's time to further connect with your inner wisdom by discovering your own experiences of physical hunger. The first two practices in this chapter introduce ways to become more familiar with the different types and levels of hunger you may experience between meals. The third practice encourages you to tune in during the course of a meal or right after a snack. And the last practice explores the differences between physical hunger and other types of messages or triggers, regardless of when they occur. These practices complement each other well, so it's fine to dive in and work with them right away. Or you can spread them out and focus on only one at a time for a few days or a week.

The Benefits of Feeling Physically Hungry

You had an introduction to understanding physical hunger in Chapter 3. Have you begun tuning in to these feelings? How does your body feel when your blood sugar is low? Does your stomach growl? Have you noticed when hunger feelings start to come back after a meal? After four hours? Six hours? You may not know the answers to those questions yet. By the time you finish the practices in this chapter, you will.

Some people experience strong and clear hunger signals. For others, these signals are much less intense. This doesn't mean, however, that you cannot become more aware of them. Or perhaps you diet so frequently—skipping breakfast, light lunch, and so on—that you spend much of the day hungry, and you've just stopped paying attention to it. Or you may be a grazer, rarely letting yourself get very hungry, out of fear or out of habit. Some people I've worked with who are grazers realize their fear of hunger started in childhood, because their parents came from families without enough food.

When I teach mindfulness of hunger to participants in the MB-EAT program, many become more aware in just a few days than they ever have been, and their appreciation and sensitivity continues to grow over time. This may take a little effort to begin to do, but can quickly become second nature. It only takes a mindful moment.

The practices in this chapter will help you:

Understand physical hunger. I know what *my* hunger feels like, but I can't tell you what *your* hunger feels like. How does your stomach feel? How does low blood sugar feel? What about if your mouth waters? Have you ever finished a substantial meal, seen a slice of your favorite pie and thought, *Maybe I'm still hungry?* Your body didn't need the pie, but your mouth still watered. You owe it to yourself to be as aware as possible of your physical hunger signals.

Know the difference between true physical hunger and other triggers to eat. Once you learn to distinguish whether or not you are truly physically hungry, you'll be able to use that information to recognize and counterbalance other triggers to eat. Rather than continue to eat automatically, you'll eat with wisdom. Soon after Marianne, one of my workshop participants, began to tune in to her physical hunger, she told me that she noticed a jittery feeling one afternoon, just before an important meeting at work. Was it hunger? Or was it nerves? After checking in, she thought, "It has been several hours since I had lunch. Yes, I am feeling stressed, but I could also use a small snack." So she ate an apple she'd brought to work, and she walked into the meeting feeling more focused and calm and less hungry. Other triggers might be particular thoughts, social events, the presence of food, or simple habit (*It's dinnertime, so I must be hungry*).

Make wiser decisions about what to eat. Tuning in to your hunger generates so much wisdom about how foods affect your body. You may notice that a sugary juice drink that caused your blood sugar to rapidly rise (and then fall) is followed again quite quickly by a return of hunger signals. Conversely, you might find that a more complex food with about the same level of calories, such as a granola bar, tends to stick with you much longer.

Have an easier time losing weight. Hunger is your body's way of telling you that it needs more nutrients. The first hints of hunger set in as blood sugar drops. If you ride out your hunger for a little while, your body will burn fuel from your fat cells, and you'll probably find that your hunger dissipates. That's wonderful. That means you're doing what your body needs you to do so you can lose weight. Eventually your hunger will increase again. When this happens, you'll know that it's time to eat.

Using the Hunger Awareness Scale

Physical hunger isn't an all-or-nothing thing. You don't go from being not at all hungry to being ravenous. The practices in this chapter will introduce you to a simple 10-point scale—with 1 being "not hungry," 5 being "moderately hungry," and 10 being "extremely hungry," and all the feelings in between. As you learn to tune in to them, you'll be able to make wiser decisions on when to eat and how much to eat. For instance, you might decide to eat a little bit an hour or so before dinner to take the edge off, perhaps reducing your hunger from an 8 to a 6. Or, you might decide that you don't need your afternoon snack just yet because, after all, you're only a 4 on your hunger scale. Hunger signals may come from your stomach but they can also come from other parts of your body. You'll learn to notice different types of signals related to different levels of hunger so you can tell when you are at a medium point of hunger, a 5 on the scale, or are only a little hungry and can wait, such as a 3. And your 3 or 7 may feel different from someone else's. It's learning to read your own experiences that's important.

As you incorporate the practices in this chapter, keep using what you've already learned. The sitting meditation will help you cultivate your ability to be mindful and become more aware of hunger experiences. The mini-meditations will bring this awareness into the moment, particularly before meals and snacks.

The Hunger Awareness Scale

To become more aware of physical hunger, you'll rate your sensations of hunger using the scale below. Some people prefer to start their scale at 0, which is fine, or to use fewer points, such as 1 to 7 or 1 to 5, but I don't recommend fewer than that. The goal is to be able to fine-tune your awareness of your hunger experiences as they move up—and down—and up again.

Not at all				Moderately					Very
1	2	3	4	5	6	7	8	9	10

Using These Practices

Practices 1, 2, and 3 guide you in tuning in to your own inner experiences of physical hunger. If you have a hard time being aware of physical hunger, then Practice 2, which guides you in letting yourself get more hungry than usual, will be particularly important to try right after Practice 1. Practice 3—observing hunger change during a meal—can wait until you've become more familiar with your own hunger signals. Finally, Practice 4 helps you begin to differentiate more between physical hunger and other feelings associated with reasons we eat. You might want to read through this practice earlier as you begin to explore hunger, but come back to it after you're more confident noticing your physical hunger signals.

PRACTICE 1

Hunger Awareness Throughout the Day

You're going to tune in to the physical sensations in your body that lead you to think you need something to eat. The longer you go between meals, the more intense your hunger will become—although it will still fluctuate. As you eat, the less intense it will become until, at some point during the meal, those feelings disappear.

The Practice: Being Mindful of Physical Hunger

The first time you do this practice, pick a time of day when you are likely to be somewhat hungry—several hours after a light meal or just before a regular mealtime. After this first time, plan to practice three to five times on a few more days, both at times when you think you are likely to be more hungry, and times when you are probably less hungry. Continue this until you become more confident that you can tune in to hunger feelings easily and quickly. But don't become frustrated if you're not always sure. Even very mindful eaters may be unsure at times.

1. **Draw your focus inward, using the mini-meditation breath awareness.** Draw on what you learned in the previous chapter. Follow your breath in and out until you feel yourself becoming more aware of your inner world. I recommend closing your eyes the first few times, until you become more easily aware of these inner experiences.

2. **Consider how hungry you feel, using the following questions as a guide.** Am I mildly hungry? Moderately hungry? Extremely hungry? Where do I feel my hunger? What does my hunger feel like? What does my stomach feel like?

What does my body feel like? Try to separate the feelings of physical hunger from any emotional hunger or food cravings going on in your mind.

3. **Using the wisdom that arises as you mindfully tune in to these feelings, note what number, from 1 to 10, best captures the level of your hunger.** There is no right answer. Remember that 1 is not hungry at all and 10 is the hungriest you've ever felt. Just notice what number comes to mind.

4. **Ask, How do I know?** Reflect what feelings in your body led you to the number you chose. How do you *know* you are a 5 or a 7 or a 3? What experiences in your body (not in your mind) told you that? Just notice these experiences. You don't have to put words to the feelings.

5. **Deepen your awareness.** As you continue to experiment with this practice, make note to yourself. What does your body feel like at different numbers? What is a 3 like? A bit of emptiness? A 6? Perhaps some stomach grumbling? An 8? Light-headed and stomach growling? Keep in mind that hunger feelings will indeed rise and fall, but when they come back, they will usually be more intense.

6. **Be aware of other triggers,** such as thoughts, feelings, or situations that lead to a desire to eat or a food craving, but when you check in, you realize you aren't really very physically hungry. Everyone will have different patterns; practice will help you learn yours.

7. **Consider also creating an Inner Craving Scale, from 1 to 10.** Craving is simply a strong desire for a particular food. How does an 8 on the craving scale feel different from an 8 on your physical hunger scale? How do you know?

Reflections on Practice 1

Tuning in to your hunger can become a quick process, a lot like becoming aware of temperature. Consider how one person might remark that a 67°F room is too cold, whereas another might say it's just right. Neither person spends a long time deciding whether he or she is cold or just right or too warm. They both just know.

Initially, it is helpful to think about tuning in to hunger regularly: before meals, during meals, after meals, and so on. Combine it with the mini-meditations you learned to do in the previous chapter. Just stop for a moment, tune in to the breath, and notice how hungry you are feeling using the 10-point scale. The more you tune in, the more your mindfulness will grow, and the easier it becomes to stop a moment and check into your hunger this way. You are now practicing a key aspect of mindful eating.

Many people ask the following questions about this and other practices in this chapter.

Is it normal to not feel hungry first thing in the morning?

I find that this experience is pretty common for many people in our programs. If this is true for you, then consider whether you may be eating too much in the evening. This is the most common time to overeat, partly because it's when we relax. But this can become a vicious circle: not eating enough during the day and then being overly hungry at night. Overeating at night carries over into the morning because, even though we digest our food while sleeping, our system is working more slowly so our blood sugar may still be high in the morning. Eating too much in the evening can be difficult to change, but one place to start is to notice the difference in the morning after you had a relatively light snack the night before versus eating quite a bit. How does that feel in your body the next day? If your stomach growls in the morning, perhaps you can applaud yourself for not having eaten too much the previous evening!

Is it ever okay to eat when I'm not hungry?

Definitely, and that's, in part, what exercising your *Power of Choice* (coming up in Chapter 12) is all about. Mindful eating is not about policing yourself with black and white rules. It's liberating. With mindful awareness of your hunger (along with many other tools), you'll be able to walk into a meeting at work, see a baked delight sitting on the table, and think, "Do I want that?" You might consider: "Am I hungry? Am I still full from lunch? Does it look amazing or only so-so? Is it a food I can get any time? Or is this going to be a special experience?" Perhaps this is the wonderful pumpkin bread that Sally brings in to the office only once a year, and you still remember it from a year ago. If so, you might decide that, yes, of course, you're going to have some pumpkin bread, even if you are not very hungry, and perhaps you can discreetly save half your slice for later in the afternoon. Rather than feeling bad about it, you'll go for it. You'll savor every bite, too.

PRACTICE 2

Allowing Yourself to Become Physically Hungry

If after a few days or a week, you've found that you've had difficulty noticing when you're physically hungry, you might try the following practice.

The Practice: Allowing Yourself to Become Hungry

1. **Pick a general time of day for this practice.** The best time of day will depend, in part, on your schedule. It also depends on your frame of mind. If you worry that you will overeat if you allow yourself to feel too hungry, then afternoon may be an optimal time for you to practice, as most people have more self-control in the afternoon than they do in the evening.

2. **Space out your meals and snacks to allow yourself to experience what true physical hunger feels like.** Have a relatively light lunch, such as a frozen meal under 300 calories, and then avoid any snacks. A frozen meal is convenient for this because you know how many calories it has, and many kinds are available at this calorie level. Then check in 3 or 4 hours after lunch. If you still don't feel hungry, then wait another hour or so. After you feel the first signals, rate your level and then try to check in about every 30 minutes and notice how the intensity or type of signal might change, perhaps delaying dinner until you're sure of these hunger experiences.

Reflections on Practice 2

If it's hard for you to be aware of physical hunger, you might keep trying this practice in different situations. You might notice how it depends on what else you are doing, how busy you are, or your mood. For example, some people feel hungrier when they're anxious, but others report losing their appetite. Or you may realize that you often get hungry in the late afternoon, perhaps because you've eaten a light lunch (see Chapter 3, Practice 3, for suggestions for working with this).

Occasionally, I work with people who resist letting themselves become hungry. They may feel anxious. Or, as mentioned earlier, they may come from families where there was often just not enough food. For them, even a little hunger seems like an emergency, one that can only be solved by eating.

If the idea of feeling hungry creates anxiety, remind yourself:

- **Physical hunger isn't a sign of weakness:** Rather it's a sign of growing awareness.
- **Some sensation of hunger is good:** Hunger can be a sign that you're losing weight!
- **You can ride the wave of hunger:** Remember, it will go up and down. You can make it through the next hour, meeting, or commute without having something to eat.
- **Hunger isn't an emergency:** After doing this practice, you can have a snack if you really want one.

PRACTICE 3

Becoming Aware of Physical Hunger Changing During a Meal

Hunger also changes throughout a meal or even during a snack. You'll understand which foods calm hunger more quickly and which ones more slowly. You'll also gain a sense of that point during a meal when hunger completely drops off.

The Practice: Becoming Aware of Hunger During a Meal or After a Snack

Use this practice regularly, throughout and even after each meal during the day:

1. **Rate your hunger just before you start eating.** Do one of your mini-meditations and check in. Where are you on the 10-point scale? How do you know?

2. **Check in again after a few bites.** Now, using another mini-meditation, how do you rate your physical hunger?

3. **Do the same a few minutes later.** And then halfway through the meal, and again at the end. Just notice how your hunger changes as the meal progresses.

4. **Once you've finished your meal, continue to practice the awareness skills you've already learned.** What if you're not sure whether you're still hungry for more food or a second helping? You might decide to wait for 10, 20, or 30 minutes, and see how your hunger feelings are then. Extend the experiences of Practice 2 and 3. Where is your hunger a few hours after a light lunch? How about after a heavy one? After a small snack? A large one?

Reflections on Practice 3

Using quick mini-meditations to tune in to subtle shifts in hunger while you're eating can be challenging, but it's very useful if you're having a multicourse meal and don't want to overeat or if you're at a party or buffet where lots of different types of delicious food are available. What does it feel like to take the edge off your hunger rather than to overeat the rolls, the salad, or an appetizer? A few carrot sticks are unlikely to change your experiences of hunger, but something with 100 to 200 calories probably will. What if you've had some nibbles at the party, but you know you're headed out to dinner later? Can you learn to notice how your hunger may have decreased from 9 or 10, and down to 5 or 6? You still want to eat something more, but you don't want to overdo it. Or perhaps those nibbles *are* dinner, and you want to bring your hunger level down further. These are important and subtle messages that can be very helpful to tune in to and use to decide what else to eat and when.

PRACTICE 4

Tune in to Physical Hunger Versus Other Urges to Eat

Once you are in the practice of pausing, tuning in to the breath, and noticing how physically hungry you are feeling using the 10-point scale, it's time to explore nonphysical hunger. We eat for many reasons in addition to physical hunger. Doing so is a normal part of everyday life. Sometimes we eat because the food is there and it appeals to us. Other times we eat because we're socializing, and everyone around us is eating too. Still other times we eat as a way of managing our emotions: to alleviate boredom, calm stress, or lift sadness. Sometimes food provides an escape, or we reach for something to eat because we're procrastinating. We'll be doing more work with these types of triggers in Chapter 13 but it's helpful to get started now noticing the range of these experiences.

The Practice: Tuning in to Other Urges to Eat

1. **Check in throughout the day and make a mental note of your other urges to eat.** By doing a mini-meditation, consider: How do I feel? How intense is my desire? What emotions, thoughts and other triggers to eat do I notice? Is it a craving for a particular food? You can also rate the strength of these desires or cravings on a 10-point scale, from "very low" to "very intense."

2. **Pay special attention to those times of day when you are unlikely to be physically hungry.** Maybe you catch yourself reaching for a snack just after lunch or dinner. You can even turn this into a detective game: "I know I'm probably not really all that physically hungry, so what else is going on? Aha! I think I'm anxious about that project (or phone call), and I'm procrastinating."

3. **And then, throughout the day, ask yourself,** "How is what I am feeling right now the same as physical hunger? Or is it different? Am I truly hungry? Or do I just want to eat for another reason?"

Reflections on Practice 4

We'll be coming back to other techniques to distinguish between physical hunger and other experiences. For now, it's important to:

- Tune in, with an attitude of curiosity and exploration.
- Start to notice your own common patterns.
- Be kind to yourself. Even if you find it easy to tune in to real physical hunger, you may be surprised for some time at

how complex the messages from your body and your mind can be.

Over time, as you use all of these practices, you'll be able to quickly tell the difference between true physical hunger and other urges to eat, such as when you realize you are actually stressed, tired, bored, or just saw the doughnuts that an office mate is eating. Or a combination of these.

Eventually you'll be able to tell how hungry you feel as quickly as you can tell how cold or tired or thirsty you feel. Soon, you'll be able to use this information to help you decide whether to eat, how much to eat, and whether to continue eating.

FAQ

I can tune in to my hunger at home, but I struggle to do it in restaurants, and I tend to order way too much. What am I doing wrong?

You're not doing anything wrong! That you can tune in at home means you are doing something right. It's easier to be aware of hunger when you're in a quiet setting, alone, and/or not distracted. A noisy restaurant is one of the most challenging places to practice hunger awareness, but it's possible! A study by Gayle Timmerman in Austin, Texas, incorporated mindful eating components and focused on helping people negotiate restaurant meals. After 6 weeks, the women had lost weight and felt much more confident about managing their eating.[1] So check your hunger before you leave for the restaurant and again before you walk in the door. Or even excuse yourself for a few quiet moments in the restroom. Feel encouraged by what you are already doing right, rather than discouraged by what you still have left to learn. In a few weeks, your mastery will grow. After all, you have many times a day to hone your awareness.

Moving On

You're now on the road to learning to tune in to a very important part of what your body and your mind has to tell you. Doing so is a core way of getting into better balance with your eating and your weight. As you learn to eat less often when you're not really hungry and learn to take the edge off your hunger without overdoing it, you may be surprised by how easy this becomes. But again, be kind to yourself. When people start to tune in, they are often surprised at how clear the signals can be some of the time, but at other times, they're relatively subtle, mixed in with all types of other messages. Keep in mind that this is normal. But as you work with the practices, you're gaining new powerful tools. You'll be able to say to yourself, and to others, "Wow, that looks really delicious, but I'm just not that hungry right now." And you'll mean it.

CHAPTER NINE

Cultivating Your Inner Gourmet

Now you're ready for some of the most pleasurable practices in this book, the very ones that will allow you to truly soak up the flavor of your favorite foods, enjoying them more than you ever have before. Let's start having fun with food and maximizing that fun by using your inner Taste Satisfaction Meter. Each of the practices in this chapter will help you learn how to savor foods that may seem particularly challenging (starting with chocolate!). They'll reawaken your confidence in being able to eat small amounts of sweet and high-fat foods.

The Benefits of Tuning In to Taste

By helping you maximize quality, the practices in this chapter will help you decrease quantity, without struggling. As you learned in Chapter 4, our taste buds are finely tuned to give us the quickest, surest feedback about whether a food is worth eating—and when we've had enough. You will also discover which foods you love and which ones you can either eat less of or don't even really like.

Once you really begin to focus on your taste experience, you will probably find that some of the foods—particularly unhealthy ones—don't taste as good as you once thought. You may become aware of chemical tastes of processed foods, of when foods are overly sweet or salty or not really possessing much of the flavor that they are advertised to have. You might end up gravitating toward some healthier options as you come to appreciate the richness of the whole grain, the lack of those underlying processed off-tastes, and the bright flavors of fresh vegetables.

Similarly, as you continually cultivate your inner gourmet, rather than experiencing some of these high-sweet, high-fat foods as addictive, you may even find that you no longer feel called to eat them at all. Until they took my workshops, many people told me, "I'm just addicted to food. As long as I am on a diet and I am not eating these foods, I'm okay. As soon as I have even a small amount, I am out of control and don't know when to stop." This all-or-nothing mind-set sets you up for psychological cravings and the false belief that you will never be satisfied unless you've eaten much more than your body needs. By allowing yourself small amounts of these very foods—and savoring them completely—you'll gain mastery over them, though with some foods more quickly than others. You may be very surprised when you really don't want more of the food you used to binge on, and you'll find that this becomes easier and easier to do.

When you become mindfully aware of taste and taste satiety, you will:

- **Know when to stop eating:** Taste awareness provides you with swift and clear messages that will help you say "enough" long before you mindlessly eat too much.

- **Stop eating foods you don't even like:** One man in our workshop ate a large Snickers bar on his work break most afternoons. Part way through the program he brought one in for a mindful eating practice that uses a favorite snack food. He took two bites and left the rest. As the group reflected on their experiences, he said, with surprise and a bit of sadness: "I don't think I like them anymore! The caramel is too sweet and the chocolate too greasy. Only the peanuts are okay—but I don't need a bar for those."
- **Stop chasing the flavor:** You're chasing the flavor when you keep eating a favorite food, especially the richer, sweeter, fattier foods, hoping to get that first exceptional taste burst back. Rather than chasing after the flavor of the first few bites, mindfulness teaches you to notice when the flavor and enjoyment wanes.
- **Gain mastery over tempting foods:** You *can* stop at a reasonable amount of any tempting food. You'll maximize your satisfaction from smaller amounts of foods just as someone might slowly sip and savor a quality glass of wine, rather than drinking it down without noticing or drinking too much altogether.

TUNING IN TO YOUR TASTE BUDS: THE TASTE SATISFACTION METER

As you practice taste awareness, you'll use a 1 to 10 meter (see page 56 for a visual) rather than the 1 to 10 scale you used for hunger awareness. Unlike a scale, a meter can fluctuate up or down, over and over again, as your mouth and mind respond to each bite.

One bite might taste amazing. Maybe it's a 9 or 10 on your meter. After several bites, however, your taste buds begin to tire and soon you are close to a 5 or 6. Then if you then take a few bites of a different food, and give your taste buds a different stimulation, perhaps you can try out that first food again, and get a few more lovely bites of pleasure—perhaps only at a 7 or 8, but still worth it. Eventually though, you will become tired of all the flavors, as your hunger and your taste buds say "enough."

You'll also notice that your taste buds tire out in two stages, if you recall from Chapter 4. The first happens relatively quickly, generally after a few bites, while the second happens after about a serving size amount of most foods. And this happens faster if you're not very hungry. At that point, you may realize you are almost not even tasting the food. What about those last few bites of a large sandwich? The whole baked potato? The 8-ounce steak? The large plate of pasta? Yes, your mouth can still probably tell what type of food it is (if you close your eyes), but unless you were very, very hungry, you might not really be tasting it much at all.

Using the Practices

The first practice uses chocolate to lay the foundation for bringing quality and enjoyment to eating. Practice 2 suggests that you cultivate your inner gourmet as you eat one of your favorite snacks. Practice 3 moves to perhaps a more challenging experience: deep-fried food. If eating this type of food feels particularly difficult, then wait until you're more confident in yourself. Practice 4 guides you into taking your inner gourmet to a full meal at a restaurant, a party, or even your own kitchen. Give yourself time to experience each practice one by one, perhaps over several weeks, and then continue practicing, engaging with your inner gourmet forever.

PRACTICE 1

Experience Chocolate Mindfully

Think back to what you experienced when you mindfully ate a few raisins in Practice 3 in Chapter 7. How did you experience this? Did each raisin taste the same as the one before? Did you find yourself feeling that you didn't want a fourth one? If you did, then you've already had a small experience of taste awareness and its power to transform your relationship with food.

For this practice, you'll use the same awareness to fully experience a sweet treat: chocolate. You might wonder: Why chocolate? Why not start with a less tempting food? You *did* start with a less tempting food—a raisin. Now you're ready to experience the power of this process with a food that may create more anxiety and more craving. That way you can truly understand just how powerful an ally your taste buds can be.

When choosing your treat, use these pointers:

- Choose a chocolate food that you find appealing and tempting, but not so much that you're unsure if you will be able to stop eating. You may wish to initially steer clear of gourmet home-baked or fresh-baked delights, choosing the less gourmet prepackaged ones instead. In my workshops, I've used store-bought brownies, Pepperidge Farm Soft Baked Captiva Dark Chocolate Brownie cookies, or a moderate-quality chocolate (such as Dove dark chocolate or milk chocolate pieces, depending on your preference).
- If you don't like chocolate, choose another type of snack food, something that you normally would think of as off limits when trying to lose weight or controlling your eating.

- Choose a simpler food over complex ones, whether chocolate or something else. If you want to use chocolate cookies, don't choose ones that also contain nuts or another flavor. The more variety of tastes and textures in a food, the longer you'll find it appealing. Eventually we'll have you work your way up to mindfully experiencing complex foods. But for this exercise, the simpler, the better.

The Practice: Experiencing Chocolate Mindfully

Once you've chosen your chocolate food, you're ready to experience it with all of your senses but especially with your taste buds. This process is similar to what you already experienced in Chapter 7 when you mindfully ate the raisins, but now you have more mindfulness experience.

1. **Place a small amount of your treat in front of you.** Make it a little more, rather than less, than you think you might want. One medium brownie or large cookie is plenty.

2. **Cut or break what you plan to eat into four to five bite-size pieces,** or use four to five small pieces of chocolate (like the Dove chocolate, which might be good for two bites, or a Hershey's Kiss).

3. **Sit in a balanced way, close your eyes, and calm yourself with a few deep breaths,** as you've already learned how to do during your mini-meditations.

4. **Open your eyes and pick up one of the pieces.** Look at this treat as if you've never before eaten it or even seen it.

What do you notice? What does it look like? Now closing your eyes, how does it smell? How does it feel when you gently touch it to your lips?

5. **Keeping your eyes closed, take one of the small pieces.** Gently hold the treat inside your mouth, resisting the urge to start chewing, and move it around with your tongue and notice how it feels and tastes.

6. **Very slowly begin to chew it, experiencing every bit of its taste.** What part of your mouth is chewing? How does the taste change as you start to chew? How high is your Taste Satisfaction Meter going? Does it change as you continue to chew this first bite?

7. **Notice the impulse to swallow.** What does that impulse feel like? It's partly just a habit. Now resist that impulse as long as you are still experiencing pleasure from this one little bite. All along the way, notice your thoughts and feelings. Are they judging the treat or judging you for eating it? When the pleasure from this little bite drops down, choose to swallow.

8. **After two to three deeper breaths, take the second piece,** again closing your eyes, smelling it, first experiencing it without chewing it, and then fully experiencing its taste and noticing where you are on the Taste Satisfaction Meter. Your meter might stay the same, go up, or go down. And again, resist swallowing it until you've extracted all the pleasure. How is it similar to the first piece? How is it different? How do the flavors linger in your mouth once

you've swallowed it? Consider that you are taking this tiny little piece of food energy into your body. Breathe.

9. **Take the third piece,** and again follow the steps. Where is your Taste Satisfaction Meter going now? How do you know? And how is this piece similar or different to the first two?

10. **With the fourth piece,** pause with your eyes open, and ask yourself if you really want to eat more. Take a moment to be aware of your breath to create a mindful space. Make a decision of whether to continue to eat. Consider how you made this decision. Are you making it because you still find the food pleasurable? Or are you attempting to chase the flavor, seeking the experience of the first bite that is no longer in your mouth? If you wish to continue eating this last piece, then lead yourself in eating it mindfully.

11. **End with bringing your awareness back to the breath.** Take two or three deeper breaths. Bring your awareness back to your body and open your eyes.

12. **Consider how this experience was similar and different to your usual way of eating.** Did the treat taste different from what you expected? Were there any surprises? What did you notice about its taste? How did it change from bite to bite? What did you notice about your thoughts and feelings as you ate?

13. **Extend your mindful awareness of the taste of this food to everything you might know about it or could find out.**

Even though this is a treat food, consider its food energy (that is, calories). How many were in the amount you ate? You might be pleasantly surprised! Consider its nutritional value (we now know that chocolate has some special health attributes). Where did the ingredients come from? Who was involved in growing and harvesting the ingredients that went into creating this little piece of pleasure? How did it come from there to your store and to you? Reflect on this awareness with curiosity and appreciation.

Reflections on Practice 1

I think you'll find that this practice will help you begin to say when you've had "enough" with conviction, so that eating feels much less like a brutal war between your desire and your willpower or self-control. You can use this practice immediately, with any food you choose to eat. Until you fully cultivate taste awareness, however, you might find that you want to stick to practicing with foods that you consider to be safer, and start with simpler foods rather than those with complex flavors. You can work up to other foods, over time, maximizing the quality of your eating experience so you can minimize the quantity.

PRACTICE 2

Experience Your Favorite Snack Mindfully

I encourage you to take at least a week or two between the chocolate practice and this one, gaining more confidence in your new relationship with your taste buds. Until now, you've been experiencing the power of using taste awareness with a sweet treat, whether chocolate or something else, and then practicing with other foods. Now, let's do the same with a favorite snack food. Maybe it's a salty and crunchy snack chip or perhaps another sweet. It's your choice. Just make it something that you think you can fully enjoy.

The Practice: Experiencing Your Favorite Snack Mindfully

You'll follow the same general procedure as you did in Practice 1.

1. **Place a small amount of your snack food in front of you.** Four or five chips or bite-size pieces are plenty.

2. **Look at your snack with fresh eyes, as if it were new to you.** What do you notice? What does it look like? Try to fully appreciate this special food.

3. **Take a small piece.** Closing your eyes, experience how it smells. How does it feel when you gently rub it along your lips?

4. **Gently place it into your mouth,** moving it around with your tongue, resisting the urge to bite down, and noticing how it feels and tastes before you start chewing. Where does it register on your Taste Satisfaction Meter?

5. **Very slowly begin chewing it, experiencing every hint of its taste.** How does the taste change as you start to chew? Where does the Taste Satisfaction Meter go now? Does it change as you continue to chew? What part of your mouth is chewing? When do you feel the impulse to swallow? What does that impulse feel like? Once you swallow, what do you continue to sense and taste?

6. **Opening your eyes just enough to pick up the next piece, follow the same process** for the second and third pieces or bites. Use awareness of your breath to create a few moments of calm space when you need it. Really enjoy these pieces, but observe the changes on the Taste Satisfaction Meter.

7. **With the fourth piece,** pause with your eyes open your eyes, and consider whether you really want to eat more. How are you making your decision? What is pulling you toward it? What is pushing you away? What thoughts, feelings, and experiences? If you decided to eat this piece, then again follow all the steps and enjoy it as much as possible. If you still have another piece, observe your desire for that piece in a similar way, and continue as you wish.

8. **Afterward, think about what you learned.** Did you discover anything new with this exercise that you didn't discover with the first one? Did you discover anything new about this very familiar food?

Reflections on Practice 2

Continue practicing with other foods you like, using your mini-meditations to continually check in. As you gain more confidence, you may wish to experience these favorite foods in a variety of settings—at home, in a restaurant, or at work. Surprisingly, a restaurant can be a safer place than home. Yes, it can be harder to focus but, on the plus side, you are being served a limited amount. You can't go back into the freezer and eat the rest of the quart of ice cream. Another option is to purchase a small amount of a favorite food—for instance, buying one cookie from a bakery—and then taking it home to eat it. Or buy a snack size container rather than a regular size box of those chips or cookies. No matter where you decide to consume your treat, really tune in to the taste and the quality of the experience. I think you'll be pleasantly surprised as that out-of-control feeling that you have often battled becomes less and less of a problem.

PRACTICE 3

Experience Your Favorite High-Fat Food Mindfully

Let's continue to explore taste awareness, this time with a crunchy, greasy food that you'd never think to eat in the name of weight loss: deep-fried food. It can be french fries or fried chicken or onion rings or something else. It's up to you.

The Practice: Experiencing Your Favorite Fatty Food Mindfully

Depending on the food you choose, you may do this at home or at a fast-food place. Give some thought to how to choose the location, the time, and how hungry you are (I recommend somewhat hungry but not starving). Also, I recommend that you do this when you are by yourself, at least the first time, as it may take some planning.

For this practice:

1. **Place a small amount of the food you've chosen in front of you.** Just a few fries or a few bites of another type of fried food will do.

2. **Follow the same sequence you did for the previous two exercises.** As you slowly savor each bite, try to notice what is so appealing about this particular food. Is it the fat? The

crunchy texture? The salt? The taste? Also try to pinpoint the point when your taste buds switch from "Wow, this is wonderful" to "Yuck, this is so greasy." Trust me, it will definitely happen. No matter what food you are eating, you will reach a point where it tastes too greasy or too salty or otherwise loses its appeal.

3. **Stop when you've reached that point.** Notice when your Taste Satisfaction Meter has dropped to where it's not really worth the calories to continue to eat. Reflect on thoughts, feelings, other experiences that arise.

Reflections on Practice 3

Begin to tune in to the varying qualities and quantities of oiliness captured by different foods: crispy vs. baked chicken, lean vs. marbled meat, high- vs. low-quality tempura (yum vs. yuck). Also consider whether the mouth feel of a higher fat food is worth the calories. If you take the skin and breading off a KFC chicken breast, you go from 350 to 140 calories. But can you still enjoy the chicken without the skin and breading? If not, then you could go ahead and have half as much of the chicken with the skin on for about the same lower calories. But some high-fat entrées add up to well over 1,000 calories. Is the taste worth the calories? Check out the Eat This, Not That[1] book series, which compares more healthy vs. less healthy foods, often at the same restaurant. The difference is virtually always due to amount of fat. They show that Cheesecake Factory Bistro Shrimp Pasta (sounds nutritious, right?) has over 2,800 calories, and 77 grams of saturated fat, whereas their Pizzette Margherita has 609, with 13 grams saturated fat.[2] What about more or less butter on popcorn, a high-oil dressing vs. a good-quality low-fat one? Or nonfat vs. low-fat vs. regular yogurt? Arby's Ham and Swiss Melt has 268 calories, with 8 grams of fat, versus the 779 calories and 45 grams of fat in the Ultimate BLT Market Fresh Sandwich. But using whole milk in your coffee instead of skim milk will only "cost" you 10 more calories for 2 tablespoons. So for some choices, the higher-fat version may shoot you past what makes sense, but for others, the difference may be negligible, for that little bit of satisfying creaminess.

PRACTICE 4

Cultivate Your Inner Gourmet Wherever You Go

Now that you've become aware of how to choose quality over quantity, try it whenever you are experiencing a food you think of as dangerous, addictive, or fattening. Try this practice with steak, alcohol, pasta, bread, or anything else that you might be afraid of overindulging on. And try it with foods that might be relatively unfamiliar to you. Especially try it when you have a variety of foods in front of you, noticing how your experience changes as you move back and forth among them.

The Practice: Experiencing Any Food Mindfully

For this practice, choose a food that is part of a meal at a restaurant, a party, or in your own kitchen. Look at your plate and choose the food that is calling to you the most, then:

1. **Begin with a mindful moment mini-meditation.** Bring yourself fully into the present, with a few deeper breaths.

2. **Experience this food through all your senses.** Visually take in the food sitting in front of you. Consider what about the food seems appealing. And then consume it using all of your senses and especially your taste buds.

3. **Chew slowly, taking note of how the taste continually changes.** Notice when the flavor begins to drop off, but pleasure still remains. Then move to one or more of the other foods you have.

4. **Return to your chosen food.** Has the pleasure increased at all? Continue eating it. When does the taste and enjoyment wear off? When does the pleasure turn into displeasure? Don't forget to combine taste awareness with tuning in to changes in your hunger as you go along. How do they interact?

5. **Give yourself permission to stop.** Put the food away or to one side. If it is appropriate, plan to ask to take the rest home.

Reflections on Practice 4

Extend this practice of focusing on a particular food by comparing the quality of similar foods. How do different types of pastas or breads compare to each other? How about different types of apples? What are the taste qualities that might make one type of beer or wine more appealing to you than another? Does the taste of one linger longer than another? Does your desire for yet another taste last longer with some foods or drinks than for others?

Try tuning in to taste awareness with complex foods, too. How long do you enjoy lasagna? Do you need a large serving? Try ice cream with treats mixed in or pizza with several toppings.

Explore how foods taste when you are very hungry and when you are moderately full. Notice how the same foods can taste different, depending on how hungry you are, and how the taste can linger for longer as well.

And notice how you do in social situations. Are you able to tune in to taste as you also talk with friends? How does socializing and other distractions help or hinder your ability to enjoy the food in front of you? Continue to experiment, applying what you've learned to a wider and wider variety of foods and situations.

During one of my workshops, one young woman excitedly shared that she'd attended a local theater opening the night before, with a reception afterward. In the past, she'd had anxiety because "there would be too many dangerous foods in plain sight," as she put it. But this night, she walked into the reception looking forward to the high-quality hors d'oeuvres they served. After a few, she found herself looking over the dessert table, telling herself she would find the one that most called to her before she left, and savor every bite of it.

As she glanced at the table, it was the peanut butter cookies that caught her eye. They looked soft, and homemade, and just like the ones her mother had made many years before.

But they were too big. So she broke off half a cookie, walked to a quiet place, and enjoyed it.

Every bite lived up to her expectations. She wanted more. So she went back to the table and picked up the other half of the cookie.

Afraid that this might lead to yet another and possibly another, she wrapped it in her napkin, and walked to her car. Getting in, she decided to have the next bite right then. That bite? It was still almost as good as the first half. The second bite? Not quite as good. And the third? There was no pleasure at all, she realized. Her taste buds had switched off. So she wrapped it back up in the napkin and put it in her purse to enjoy the following day.

To her surprise on the following day, she still didn't want any more of it. So, eventually, she threw it away, appreciative of the cookie but feeling victorious. It seems that part of her taste experience had been the excitement of old memories. But without that excitement, the taste fled. I've had that experience myself, with the first few bites of a family dessert at the holidays or a special appetizer at a restaurant. Would I enjoy it as much if I had it again right away? Probably not.

FAQ

Do I always have to engage my inner gourmet?

No, you don't. After all, not every morsel is gourmet, and not all foods are worth eating slowing and mindfully. There will be times when you've stopped at a convenience store during a road trip and, though you've chosen the best the store had to offer, your meal—whether it's a sandwich or a cereal bar—isn't worth savoring slowly. You're merely eating it for the food energy, little more. Or you've really enjoyed the first half of the sandwich, but you know you need the rest of it to get you through the afternoon, even though the taste has diminished; what's more, you can't really wrap it up to finish later. There are many different elements of being mindful. You might decide that it's not worth being all that mindful of a food's flavor, but it is still worth being mindful of your hunger and fullness signals or how much food energy you consume.

Moving On

The more you practice, the more you'll develop your inner gourmet, and the more automatic it will be to tune in to taste awareness, enjoying your food more yet noticing the exact point when a particular food loses its appeal. You may also notice, as did the woman with the peanut butter cookie, that taste satiety can carry over to the next day! You'll also become more discerning, realizing that some foods simply are not really worth eating, except perhaps as fuel. And as you learn to savor more nutritious foods, without preservatives, you may also realize that the taste begins to appeal more and more. But as with other mindful eating practices, tuning in to taste satisfaction and taste satiety and using them to help create a more balanced and flexible approach to eating will evolve over time.

FAQ

Does tuning in to my inner gourmet mean that I always have to eat slowly?

No, it doesn't. As you connect more mindfully with your eating, you'll find you can move back to eating at a completely usual pace and still tune in to your taste experience. This also isn't another "should"! It's just another powerful tool to help you savor your meals and snacks without overeating.

CHAPTER TEN

Eating Just the Right Amount

Now that you've spent some time becoming acquainted with your inner gourmet, let's explore additional feedback signals that help us decide when we've eaten enough. We've all experienced that uncomfortable "I can't believe I ate the whole thing" sensation. While it might seem as if that stuffed sensation arises quickly and without warning, this isn't the case. As you've just learned, your taste buds provide an early sign of satisfaction, sometimes just a few bites into a snack or meal, but your body may still not feel satisfied. In this chapter, you'll learn how to become aware of the two additional processes that were introduced in Chapter 4:

- **Stomach fullness:** This is what you feel in and around your stomach based on the weight and volume of what you've eaten, and how quickly it moves on out of your stomach.

- **Body satiety:** This is the sense of energy and well-being—or tiredness and bloating—that sets in as blood sugar rises and various biochemicals shift. While it might be considered the opposite of hunger—as some of the same processes are involved—it's useful to tune in to it separately. It starts to happen fairly quickly, but may continue to grow for a while, as food is slowly digested.

One woman in a workshop often overate when she had a snack, thinking that she needed a large amount of food in order to feel sated. After becoming mindfully aware of fullness and satiety, though, she found that she could often limit herself to a small granola bar and, just 10 minutes later, notice the improvement in her sense of well-being, without becoming uncomfortable as she usually did.

The Benefits of Paying Attention to Fullness and Satiety

If we ate to excess only a few times a year—perhaps during big family celebrations such as Thanksgiving—eating overly large portions wouldn't really be a problem. Overeating a few times a year isn't what leads to weight gain, and it isn't what stops you from weight loss either.

It's overeating on a regular basis that does it. Once you tune in to these feelings of fullness and satiety, you'll be better able to finish meals feeling satisfied but not stuffed. You'll also:

Have an easier time losing weight. If you routinely eat past the point of comfort, whether a little or a lot, you're continually taking in more calories than your body needs and will slowly gain weight, rather than lose it. Or else you'll keep on alternating dieting (being good) with bingeing (being bad). By tuning in to fullness and satiety, you gain more awareness, which will help you stop eating before you've eaten too much, whether it's a lower calorie, bulkier food or a high-energy, easily absorbed food that you might have almost always eaten too much of in the past.

You'll feel more satisfied, and you'll feel it sooner. Body satiety can happen in a matter of minutes. My husband has diabetes. He can go from feeling light-headed and shaky to feeling fine a few minutes after eating a cookie or two or drinking some juice. The changes probably won't be as dramatic for you, but if you tune in, you'll more easily notice shifts in your body sooner after starting to eat.

You'll stop before too much. Eating past the point of comfort is very common. We might override an earlier point of satisfaction because we don't want to waste food or someone is pressuring us to eat, eat, eat or think we will feel content only if we eat to a high level of fullness. This chapter will help you finish meals feeling satisfied but not sluggish or bloated.

Everyone can learn how to tune in. These are mindfulness skills that you can learn and develop quickly. No matter how out of control your eating has seemed or overweight you are, you can definitely become aware of your inner sensations of fullness and of your overall sensations of body satiety or satisfaction. For some people, the process of tuning in is easier than it is for other people, but I've never worked with someone who couldn't do it at all.

The 10-Point Fullness Scale

You'll become aware of fullness in much the same way you became aware of your hunger: by using a 10-point scale. Number 1 on the scale is "not full at all," and 10 is "completely full." "Moderately full" or "full enough" varies from person to person, but it's probably around 6 or 7. That's when your stomach feels a little distended. You might not want to go out and do heavy exercise, but you'd be fine going for a walk without feeling uncomfortable.

You'll use your fullness scale in conjunction with your hunger scale. As you eat, your hunger goes down and your fullness goes up. As the span of time lengthens after eating, your fullness goes down and your hunger goes up. That said, the two scales are not merely two ends of a continuum; they represent different processes in the body and the brain.

As you can see from the illustration below, they overlap. For example, because of this overlap, it's possible to have a small snack and feel less hungry but not yet full at all.

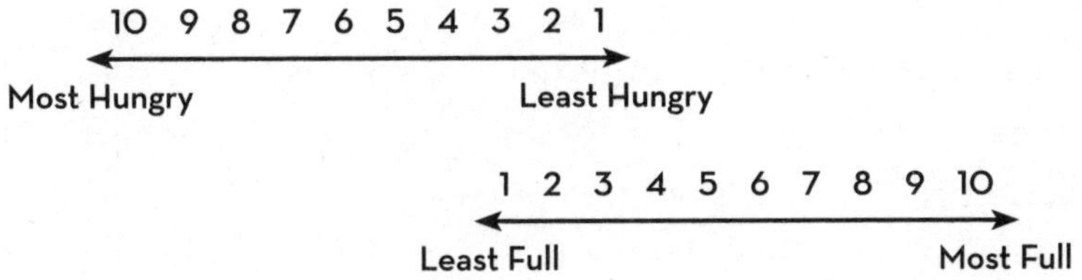

10 9 8 7 6 5 4 3 2 1

Most Hungry ←→ Least Hungry

1 2 3 4 5 6 7 8 9 10

Least Full ←→ Most Full

Using the Practices

The first practice, drinking a large amount of water fairly quickly, will help you use the 10-point fullness scale to tune in to the differences between feelings of stomach fullness and body satiety. Both of these feelings are helpful for getting into better balance with how much you're eating, so you want to be able to tune in to them separately. The second practice focuses on body satiety, using the same 10-point scale but with the focus only on body satiety. Give yourself a few days to notice the experiences from Practice 1 and then move on to Practice 2. You'll find you can use the experience from both practices many times a day.

PRACTICE 1

Drinking a Large Bottle of Water

This practice will help you learn the difference between stomach fullness (a growing tightness and fullness in your abdomen) and body satiety (the energy and well-being that sets in as nutrients flood the bloodstream). When you drink a lot of water, you fill your stomach and weigh it down. But because water contains no nutrients, it doesn't affect your blood sugar, so will give you a sense of what full means, separate from any food value.

To do the practice, use a 16- or 20-ounce bottle of water or fill a clear container or two large glasses with about this total amount of water. Find a time to do this practice when you haven't eaten for at least several hours. You might also want to let yourself get somewhat thirsty, but that's not necessary. It just helps your mind and body feel more excited about drinking all that water. It's important to drink the water fairly quickly so it stays in your stomach. It will be uncomfortable—but that's the intention.

The Practice: How You'll Drink the Water

Once you have your glasses or bottle of water:

1. **Close your eyes.** Take a few deep breaths, and center your mind by doing a mini-meditation.

2. **Notice your sensations of stomach fullness.** On the 1 to 10 scale, how full does your stomach feel before you start?

Become aware of all of the sensations that have helped you know your rating of fullness.

3. **Drink half of your bottle of water or one of your glasses of water.** Do this fairly quickly.

4. **Tune in again.** How full are you on the same 1 to 10 scale? Has your rating changed? What sensations are you experiencing to change your rating?

5. **Quickly drink the rest of the water**—or as much as you possibly can.

6. **Tune in and again rate your level of fullness using the same scale**. How has it changed? How did drinking the water affect your level of fullness?

Reflections on Practice 1

You'll probably find, as many of my workshop participants have done, that drinking this much water causes you to quickly feel uncomfortable. That's precisely the point. And if you compare the amount of water to regular food (2 to 2½ cups), it's about the total of a bowl of soup, a couple of rolls, and a small salad. With practice, you'll be able to notice your sense of stomach fullness earlier during meals, too.

As you begin bringing this awareness to regular eating experiences, you might find that you prefer to describe your level of fullness as "somewhat full," "moderately full," and "very full." Some people love the 1 to 10 scale and take to it quickly, saying things like, "When I was half way through lunch, I was a 5, but then I kept eating until I got to a 7." For others, the difference between 6 and 7 or 3 and 4 just isn't large enough to notice, and that's okay. In the beginning, the 1 to 10 scale can help you tune in to subtle gradations in your fullness, helping you see that you don't automatically go from empty to stuffed right away. Once you are able to tune in to the body feelings you're having, that's all the personal awareness you need.

As you try out this practice during your regular meals, you may realize certain patterns. Sometimes my clients will tell me, "I always eat to a 10." Do you eat to a 10 when you have breakfast? Or a snack? No, you probably stop eating much sooner, and you still feel satisfied. You can do the same for all of your meals. As you become more and more practiced, you might even challenge yourself to decide on your desired level of fullness ahead of time. For instance, if you are having a snack, you might decide you want to eat only to a level of fullness on the lower end of your scale—a 2, 3, or 4, perhaps. If you are sitting down to dinner, on the other hand, you might decide to finish the meal at a higher level of fullness, perhaps a 6 or a 7, and about the same place for overall satiety/satisfaction. But try to do this with a sense of exploration, curiosity, and flexibility, and not as a way to police yourself.

Marie, a participant in one of my mindful eating groups who had had a pattern of binge eating several days a week, shared how disappointed she was that she'd eaten to a 7 when she'd set out to eat to a 5. There was a moment of silence. And then another woman spoke up and said, "Marie, in one week you've learned to tell the difference between a 5 and a 7. That's amazing!"

PRACTICE 2

Tune In to Your Body Satiety by Enjoying a Small Treat

Now that you have gained some awareness of your sensations of stomach fullness, you're ready to learn how to pay attention to your sense of body satiety. For this practice, you'll choose a small snack to eat. It should be small enough *not* to weigh down and expand your stomach by very much. It should also be composed mostly of fast-digesting sugar. That way it will raise your blood sugar quickly, causing you to notice a growing sense of body satiety within 5 or 10 minutes. A candy bar, a couple of cookies, or a glass of orange juice are all options. You might aim to have the full amount add up to 150 to 200 calories. *Note:* If you have diabetes, you might be able to skip this practice, because, as mentioned earlier, you probably already know what it's like to take in this type of food when your blood sugar is low.

Consume your treat during a time of day when you feel somewhat hungry, perhaps several hours after your last meal but not just before your next meal.

The Practice: How to Enjoy Your Snack

1. **Place the snack food in front of you.** Close your eyes and do a mini-meditation.

2. **Once you feel aware, notice sensations in your body.** On the 1 to 10 scale, how physically hungry do you feel? How do you know that? Become aware of all of the sensations that have helped you to arrive at your rating.

3. **Then eat or drink about half of the snack.** Immediately after you eat, check your level of fullness. But then, unlike for the water, wait for at least 5 minutes, preferably for 10 minutes, before coming back to eat more. You can do something else during this time, but you might want to set a timer so you don't forget to check in.

4. **Tune in again.** Use a mini-meditation to consider how your energy level, mood, and sense of well-being have changed. How has your hunger changed? How full do you feel on the 10-point scale? Can you notice any feelings related to body satiety, on the same 1 to 10 scale? Keep in mind these are not the same things. You might notice more satiety as the sugar energy is absorbed, but less fullness as the snack or liquid moves beyond your stomach. What sensations caused you to change your rating from immediately after eating?

5. **Then consume the rest of the snack.** Remain mindful of the sensations you feel in your body.

6. **Tune in over the next 5 to 10 minutes and again rate your level of fullness and your body satiety using the same scale.** How have they changed? How has this small amount of food affected your sense of well-being, mood, and overall sense of satisfaction? How are these feelings different from each other? What about in 20 minutes?

Reflections on Practice 2

What have you learned? Do you now feel that you can explore the difference between fullness and body satiety? How about the difference between body satiety and other sensations, such as tiredness or boredom? If you found the differences in these feelings were too subtle, try this with a larger amount of food. Body satiety may still be clearest after a larger meal, about 20 minutes (or longer) after you finish eating. Fullness may be diminishing, as food moves out of your stomach, but body satiety may still be strong—and it's not just the opposite of no hunger. Keep practicing. Over time, you'll get better and better at telling the difference.

PRACTICE 3

Explore the Effects of Different Types of Foods on Fullness and Body Satiety

Choose three foods that have approximately the same amount of food energy (or calories). Between 250 and 300 calories is a good goal. Choose foods that vary substantially in their fiber, sugar, and nutrient balance.

Three possibilities for this practice:

- **High fiber:** A fairly large amount (5 to 6 cups) of lightly buttered microwave popcorn. *Note:* Theater popcorn with butter is *much* higher in calories than this for the same amount, so use a home-popped type with listed calories.
- **High sugar:** A large (20 ounce) bottle of juice. *Note:* You do *not* have to drink it quickly, as you did in Practice 1.
- **High complexity:** A healthy food entrée that includes a protein source. As noted earlier, frozen meals are convenient because the calories are clearly identified, and readily available at this calorie level.

You could also put together a combination of foods that you prefer as long as you calculate and compare the caloric levels of each.

You'll complete your practice over a span of three days, experimenting with one food each day to see how it affects your levels of stomach fullness and satiety. Each day, practice at approximately the same time of day, perhaps at lunch or later afternoon, at a time when you are moderately hungry *and* have the flexibility of going without eating for another couple of hours. This will allow you time to fully evaluate the effects of what you've just eaten. If you can't do this three days in a row, try to do it within a week. Otherwise, you might find it hard to remember and compare the feelings experienced from each food.

Practice 3: How to Explore Different Foods

1. **Check in by using a mini-meditation just before eating.** Rate your levels of hunger, fullness, and body satiety.

2. **Eat or drink half of the food.** As you eat, you can check in with your taste satisfaction, but for this exercise, it shouldn't determine whether you continue or not. Then check in again in 5 minutes, taking time to rate your hunger, fullness, and sense of body satiety and consider how you arrived at your ratings.

3. **Finish your meal.** Again, tune in and rate your hunger, fullness, and body satiety after another 5 or 10 minutes. Then continue to check in over the next 1–3 hours. You might jot down notes to remind yourself of your insights.

On the following day, complete the same process with the second food choice. On the third day, do this with the final option.

Reflections on Practice 3

If you used popcorn, did you find that it left you feeling quite full initially, that it didn't affect your body satiety as much, and that your hunger came back fairly quickly, within an hour or two? Similarly, perhaps the large glass of juice might not have lasted even as long as the popcorn, but a certain sense of well-being might have increased right away—or perhaps you just craved more food. On the other hand, the chicken breast, brown rice, and vegetables in the frozen meal may have led to a lower level on your fullness scale, but kept you sated for longer than did the popcorn. The meal contains the same food energy (number of calories) as the other choices but offers a more complex range of nutrients, and the different components of the meal take different amounts of time to digest.

PRACTICE 4

Full Meals: Don't Eat Everything on Your Plate

As your awareness of fullness and satisfaction increases, you're bound to encounter times when you think you've had enough, but you feel compelled to go on eating. Whenever this happens, try to become aware of what's behind your urge to continue eating. Do you feel pressured by someone to eat more? Or perhaps you just don't want to disappoint the cook. Have you fallen into the "I've blown it, I might as well keep on going" mind-set trap, or do you feel uncomfortable wasting food?

The Practice: How to Be Okay with Leaving Food on Your Plate

1. **Intentionally serve yourself more than you think you want to eat.**

2. **As you eat, practice everything you've already learned.** Remain aware of your changing sense of hunger, fullness, and taste satisfaction.

3. **Once you feel you've eaten enough, stop eating.** Put your utensils down, but give yourself permission to have more in 5 or 10 minutes if your body is suggesting you do so.

4. **Consider your thoughts and emotions.** What thoughts are running through your mind? If you feel some resistance, consider where that sensation is coming from.

5. **Wrap up the rest of your meal to enjoy later on.** Or, you might scrape it into the compost. It's your choice.

Reflections on Practice 4

I think you'll find, as do so many of my workshop participants, that the urge to go on eating often has a lot less to do with body satisfaction and more to do with those old rules that are still functioning mindlessly. Where do you feel these beliefs come from? Chances are they were instilled in you during childhood when your parents told you to always clean your plate. How have these beliefs affected your awareness, enjoyment, and body size? Such beliefs are not helpful at all, are they? Consider these ways to shift your thinking.

If you've already had enough at a meal, just three more bites of the main course, the side dishes, and dessert can still add up to a hundred calories or more, or almost 10 pounds of the weight you wish you could lose, if you do this day after day, meal after meal. Toss it or save it. Those small amounts may not be enough for a full meal, but put together over several days, could be combined for a satisfying lunch. And you'll likely enjoy them more later, than simply stuffing them in now.

When you are served more at a restaurant than you need to feel satisfied, remind yourself that you will get *more* value out of packing up leftovers to eat the following day than you will by cleaning your plate. You may also get more enjoyment from it a day or two later, too.

Even if you can't bring food home or save it for later, ponder what's more of a waste: having extra food eventually go into the compost and create rich soil for a garden *or* eating hundreds of calories you don't need and will not enjoy? What do you gain by eating more than you need?

If you feel bad that the chef will see the uneaten food on your plate and think you did not enjoy your meal, consider that chefs plate meals for the average patron. Some have huge appetites, others very small ones, and many others somewhere in between the two. The chef has no idea how much food your body needs or how hungry you are. Ask the waiter to compliment the chef for you—and don't worry about the food going back.

If you're worried about hurting someone else's feelings, think creatively. Many of my clients feel especially challenged when having a meal with relatives who encourage them to keep eating. Some have gotten around this issue by telling white lies, "I'm so sorry. This is great, but I had a late lunch and I'm really not so hungry." Others have only a small serving, but ask to take some home to have later, when they are hungry and can truly enjoy it. Whichever method you use, try to be complimentary, gracious, and firm. Make it clear that your refusal has nothing to do with the food being served or with the person serving it.

When you have access to an all-you-can-eat bargain buffet, shift your focus away from "getting the most food for your buck" and toward giving yourself permission to "play with your food" (something your parents probably told you *not* to do). Rather than eating as much as possible, see this as an opportunity to sample small amounts of many different items. In Chapter 12, you'll explore more how to do this.

You might find that some situations are more challenging than others. As your awareness grows, you'll be able to check into these yourself more and more easily, and you'll come up with your own ways to shift your thinking.

Moving On

If you haven't done so already, this is a great point in the program to revisit the Circle of Being and the Keep It Off Checklist you filled out in Chapter 6. I think you'll be pleased by how much progress you've already made.

As you cultivate your ability to know the difference between hunger and overall satiety and how the two overlap and work together to help you make eating decisions, you'll become more attuned to how these experiences vary with different types of food. You'll also become more aware of how levels of hunger, fullness, and satiety affect your decisions about what and how much to eat.

As you did with your hunger awareness practices, you'll find it much easier to tune in to fullness and other satiety signals when you are undistracted. There may even be some situations when you struggle to be aware of your growing sense of fullness or satiety at all. Don't give up. Just keep practicing, becoming mindful of which distractions—the television, a darkened movie theater, a lively conversation—pull your attention so much that pairing them with food just not might be worth it.

For example, I find that's true for popcorn at the movies. I'd rather devote my attention to just one or the other. Some of my clients, however, tell me that the entire movie experience isn't the same without the popcorn. So they now go into the movies knowing that they'll likely finish the whole bucket. So they take that into account, and order a smaller bucket, with less butter. Sometimes they substitute this for dinner or at least eat less for dinner. You might decide the same.

CHAPTER ELEVEN

Calories: Turning Off the Panic Button

Now that you've been creating the foundation for the inner wisdom of mindful eating, you're ready to begin linking these together with outer wisdom, particularly how to relax about creating a healthier balance of food and being realistic about how much you choose to take in, with less struggle and self-judgment.

Perhaps you have an on-again, off-again relationship with calories. Perhaps, when you have attempted to lose weight, you've been hypervigilant and kept track of every single one of them. And when you're not trying to lose weight, it may be the opposite. And, sometimes, you feel you'd rather not know. So it's understandable that just thinking about calories might make you feel anxious, and even question whether tuning in to calories in foods can be part of mindful or balanced eating.

But calories are nothing to fear. They're just the energy stored inside a food that your body needs. Some foods contain more energy than others, but most foods are not inherently good or bad in smaller quantities or inherently fattening or slimming, at least not in the context of an overall healthier balance of foods. Developing your understanding of food energy will help you ease anxiety about calories. It will also help you make more informed decisions, giving you another powerful tool in your mindfulness kit.

The Benefits of Food Energy Awareness and Balance

When you develop an awareness of food energy, outer wisdom starts to combine with inner wisdom, to help you:

- **Uncover hidden sources of weight gain.** As I noted earlier, not knowing the food energy of what you are eating is like trying to stick to a budget without keeping an eye on prices. By knowing more about the food energy contained in various meals and foods, you'll make decisions that help you eat less and that support weight loss rather than getting in the way.
- **Avoid becoming too hungry and then overeating.** You'll know how much to eat to prevent the late afternoon or early evening munchies that might lead to an entire evening of overeating.
- **Create an eating plan that includes the foods you love.** Instead of depriving yourself by declaring many of your favorite foods off limits, which often backfires, you'll be able to truly enjoy your favorite foods—and eat less of them.
- **Find ways to increase your activity level (burn more**

calories) that are satisfying, rewarding, and feasible to maintain. You can increase your metabolism and feel healthier by investing only a few hours per week. You can look for ways to build in more activity (think stairs rather than elevator). Use a pedometer to first check your usual daily walking—then to increase your steps by 10 to 20 percent each week. Try out some fitness classes to find one you like. Give yourself a year to experiment with different plans. And be careful not to fall prey to the *compensation effect* ("I worked out, so I can have that second helping").

You'll find that I'm not going to give you a single straightforward rule to follow. Yes, given the same amount of activity and exercise, you must consume less food energy if you wish to lose weight, but you can be in charge of what you cut or shrink from your eating plan. The key to using your outer wisdom is not to blindly follow the rules of one diet over another. Rather, it's to think about how information applies to you and to combine it with the inner wisdom tools you've already learned. So, yes, dry toast has fewer calories than heavily buttered toast, but is it satisfying? Do you want it?

What about toast with a little jam? Or using half as much butter? How do you find the right intersection of fewer calories and more enjoyment? What are you willing to change in your eating, not for one week or one month, but permanently? That intersection is where inner wisdom and outer wisdom meet, and it's where you'll be happiest.

In that way, it's not just knowledge. You are cultivating wisdom.

The practices in this chapter will help you develop a sense of curiosity and exploration regarding all those possible choices. They are designed to help you move away from the food police mentality, toward simply seeing nutritional information as something you can use, allowing you to make more balanced choices.

FAQ

I don't even want to think about counting calories. I want to put that behind me. Can I still follow this program?

Rather than think of this approach as a way to diet or as a form of restriction, think of it as a way to bring wisdom to your eating. You are not counting calories. You are gathering information to help you make choices. This is about being flexible, giving yourself both the nutritional value and the pleasure you deserve without beating yourself up about it. It's about enjoying smaller amounts of the foods you love, while incorporating other food options that may be surprisingly substantial, yet without breaking your food energy budget. You could even try to switch off your deprivation mind-set completely. As noted earlier, rather than seeing 1,800 or 2,000 calories per day (on average) as something you have to limit yourself to, how about seeing that amount as something you get to "spend"? Now let yourself think about the most satisfying yet balanced ways to do that.

Using the Practices

These practices are designed to help you develop your outer wisdom and then apply it to your own food choices. Practice 1 provides a foundation, beginning with your own kitchen, to inform yourself about the food energy in your favorite foods. This links well with Practice 2, the 500-Calorie Challenge. You'll find that Practice 3, spreading out your food energy, meshes really well with learning to manage feelings of hunger during the day. And use Practice 4 to make food choices that balance nutritional and health needs with your inner gourmet. You'll learn to see calorie counts in a new way and begin to get more comfortable with choosing healthier foods, while feeling more truly satisfied by what you eat.

PRACTICE 1

Explore Your Kitchen Cupboards

Before you can apply outer wisdom, it's important to expand your knowledge about the energy inside various foods. One of the easiest ways to do this is to explore your own kitchen.

The Practice: Exploring Your Kitchen

With a sense of adventure and curiosity, check out what you already have on hand in your cupboards.

1. **Pull boxed and bagged foods off the shelf, and take a look at their Nutrition Facts labels.** The Nutrition Facts label lists the calories, calories from fat, total fat, cholesterol, and other nutritional contents of the food you are eating. For this practice, you need to focus in only on the serving size, the servings per container, and the number of calories per serving.

2. **Try to do this with a sense of exploration.** This isn't about judging yourself for the types of foods you find. Again,

think of the calorie information in the same way you might think about a price tag. You don't judge clothes as good or bad depending on their price. Similarly there's no reason to do the same with food. This isn't about saying some foods are off limits. Rather, it's about gaining insight into how much you can afford to consume, and it's about taking the foods you love out of the off-limits category and putting them back into the on-limits one. You might be surprised. You're going to find that some of the foods you love actually have fewer calories than you thought, especially in smaller amounts than the listed serving size.

3. **Try to find five foods that have fewer calories than you might assume in the amounts that you would find satisfying.** Maybe two scoops of ice cream is a lot, but what about ½ cup? Or a ¼ cup? The whole bag of corn chips is too much, but one full serving, poured into a bowl, might be just right—or better yet, what about eating only a few mindfully?

4. **Conversely, look for some surprises in the other direction.** Try to find at least three seemingly healthy foods that contain more calories than you might think. Many people fall prey to the "healthy food" effect, consuming larger servings of healthy foods because they assume these foods are lower in calories than those with fewer nutrients. For instance, many people think of trail mix as a healthy snack and, as a result, may graze on it as if it were low calorie. But a 160-calorie serving of a typical trail mix is just 3 tablespoons. Even for a small snack, I don't

know many people who feel satisfied on just 3 tablespoons. So take a look at the labels for dried fruit, packaged bars and muffins, granola, veggie crisps, and whatever else you have on hand and see if you come up with any surprises.

5. **After you sleuth around your kitchen, expand your food energy knowledge even more by trying this same exercise in your local grocery store**, and by carefully looking at the food energy information supplied by restaurants (if you live in an area that requires this). Another fun resource is the Eat This, Not That series of books, which lay out surprising examples of foods either higher or lower in calories than you might have expected. But even here, you could consider how the foods they mention line up if you eat half a serving, rather than the full amount.

6. **Continue to look for surprises in both directions.** Consider the following: Can I be satisfied on the recommended amount? Is there an amount that would satisfy me and still not overwhelm my food energy budget for the day? Is it worth eating this food in this amount? Or will I usually wish I'd had more?

Reflections on Practice 1

Were there surprises in both directions? When I do this exercise in my workshops, there always are. Many of my workshop participants mistakenly assume that the cheese and crackers we offer them to help develop taste awareness are loaded with calories. When I ask them to guess the number of calories in each one, I get all sorts of answers, ranging from 30 calories to 60 calories (and occasionally more) a piece. Yet this is just one Wheat Thin with a small square of cheese on it. Each one contains about 20 calories (about 9 from the cracker and 11 from the cheese). Many workshop participants find that they feel quite satisfied with just three of these when they consume them mindfully, even exclaiming, "Wow, I can eat cheese and crackers again!" This is, of course, totally different from mindlessly eating half the box of crackers and the whole block of cheese in front of the TV or during a binge when you're angry about something. That could easily total 1,000 calories or more, depending on how much you consume.

On the other end of the spectrum, one of my clients checked into the bran muffin she ate each morning. The muffin was loaded with nuts, dried fruit, shredded carrots, and even zucchini. It certainly sounded healthier than what she truly wanted: a doughnut. Yet, when she explored the food energy cost, she was surprised. The muffin contained 450 calories, whereas the doughnut had about half that. For about a week she treated herself to doughnuts. After that she found she had tired of them and wanted the more complex flavors of the muffin. So she started eating only half of each muffin, keeping the rest for the next day (saving both calories and money).

As you expand your knowledge, you'll probably run up against some of the same questions I hear from my workshop participants.

How can I find out how many calories a food or a meal contains?

When you want to know the calories of unpackaged foods such as produce or of various dishes you are considering ordering in a restaurant, you have several options:

- **Look online.** Many different apps, online services, and websites will provide you with the nutritional data on a variety of foods and meals. CalorieKing (CalorieKing.com) is a reliable source of information. So is the U.S. Department of Agriculture's (USDA) SuperTracker: Food-a-Pedia (supertracker.usda.gov). Many restaurant chains are now required to post calories on their menus (and others post them online).

- **Buy a calorie-counting guide.** These booklets list hundreds of foods. Carry your guide with you so you can easily consult it wherever you go. The CalorieKing guide is comprehensive and the one we use in our program.
- **Invest in a set of measuring cups and a small food scale.** It can be very hard to judge portion sizes. How much breakfast cereal equals ¼ cup, ½ cup, or 1 cup? How much does your cereal bowl actually hold? If the serving size is ½ cup and you mindlessly pour yourself 1 cup, you're consuming twice as many calories. The serving size for other foods is defined by ounces, so you need a small food scale to measure these—it can be hard to judge the difference between 2 and 4 ounces. This is true of all foods, and most of us need tools to guide us. The point is not to become obsessive about using these, but simply to have them on hand to inform yourself.
- **Make educated guesses.** Certain types of foods contain roughly the same number of calories. So, for instance, you don't necessarily need to know the calorie count of every single vegetable or every single cut of meat. As long as you know the information in the following chart, you'll be able to make fairly accurate guesses.

Type of Food	Serving Size	Looks Like . . .	Calories per Serving
Nonstarchy vegetables (lettuce, tomatoes, celery and so on)	1 cup raw (½ cup cooked)	Baseball	25
Root vegetables (potatoes, yams)	3 ounces (½ medium potato)	Size of a computer mouse	80
Legumes (beans, lentils, black eyed peas)	½ cup	Tennis ball	115
Fruit	1 piece of whole fruit, ½ a grapefruit, or 1 cup berries or cubed melon	Baseball	60
Protein (poultry, meat or fish)	3 ounces	Checkbook or deck of cards	Lean = 100 Medium fat = 150 High fat = 220
Fats (butter, oil, mayo)	1 teaspoon	Tip of your thumb	34
Sugar	1 teaspoon	Tip of your thumb	15

Should I always stick to the serving size listed on a package?

When deciding what amount to eat, combine your outer wisdom (calories per serving) with inner wisdom (How hungry am I? What would satisfy me?) and then exercise your Power of Choice. On the one hand, it's okay to eat more than one serving of a food at a time if that is your choice. Just be honest with yourself. A very large apple may have double the calories of a small apple. If you consume 1 cup of granola instead of ½ cup, you are consuming twice as many calories. On the other hand, 1 cup boxed pasta or rice is usually a serving and has about 200 calories, but perhaps you don't really want that much. You may find ½ cup of creamy bottled Alfredo sauce is about 200 calories, but ¼ cup of the light variety is only 60—so enjoy!

Or using your inner gourmet, you may find that you are satisfied with far less than the serving size. Savoring just three bites of something would rarely be as much as the listed serving size. A few crackers with a little cheese is far less than the 14 to 16 crackers often identified as a serving, which equals 140 calories. Or savor two squares of a gourmet chocolate bar at about 60 calories, rather than the 190 identified as a serving.

PRACTICE 2

The 500-Calorie Challenge

In the past, when you've dieted, you've probably restricted your eating using external limits that were created by someone else. Maybe, based on the diet you were following, you consumed 1,200 to 1,400 daily calories. And you probably gave up certain foods, especially those that were high on your craving list. In both ways, you were probably left with a sense of not being allowed to eat what you wanted or as much as you wanted. In the short term, this might have felt like a relief, as the rules of the diet helped kick in your willpower. But after that came fear, anxiety, and struggle because the diet didn't teach you how to be flexible or manage moderation.

The 500-Calorie Challenge is different. In this practice, you'll remove up to 500 calories from your daily eating by deciding for yourself what to still eat and what not to eat. The 500 calories is just a rough goal and is the maximum number of calories I recommend cutting back on at any one time. Not everyone needs to remove this many calories. If your weight loss goal is in the range of 20 to 30 pounds, then I recommend looking for 200 to 300 calories to remove, as 500 calories is likely too much. That's still enough to result in losing a couple of pounds per month and may better reflect your long-term food energy (caloric) needs. Alternatively, if you have more than 50 or 60 pounds to lose, after a few months working with (and meeting) the first 500-Calorie Challenge, and if your weight loss has plateaued, you might want to find another few hundred unneeded calories to work with.

The important thing is this: You are in charge. This is about thinking carefully about the food energy you can remove, quite possibly without missing it much at all. You'll shift your mind-set away from "I can't have this," and over to "How much of this do I really need to feel satisfied?" So you won't be left with that sense of rebellion or yearning that you've probably experienced in the past, because you'll choose to reduce or eliminate foods that you can truly live without.

The Practice: The 500-Calorie Challenge

You'll start this challenge over one week and then continue it over the following weeks. Be sure to choose the first week as a time that is fairly typical for you—not a vacation week, one with visitors, or frequent eating out (unless that's what you usually do). During the first week, the goal is to simply take note of ways that, on average, you might remove about 500 calories (or your chosen goal) from your daily intake *but without making these changes.* Consider finding more possibilities than just what adds up to 500 calories. This will give you more options in case one or more of the changes you try to make turns out to be harder than you expected.

1. **Think about what you usually eat,** both at home and when you dine out.

2. **Look for ways to remove up to 500 calories a day from what you eat** by identifying between 5 and 10 foods (or

more) that you could omit or serving sizes that you could cut down. What happens, for instance, if you switch from full-fat mayo to low-calorie mayo or from regular salad dressing to low-calorie dressing? How many calories would that save you each day? Or instead of 1 tablespoon of butter you use 1 teaspoon? What if, instead of 1 cup of ice cream at night, you have ½ cup? Or savor only a few spoonfuls? What if you consume one fewer soft drinks a day or order the small fries rather than the large? Or what if you share your fries or burger with someone?

3. **Keep using the 500-Calorie Challenge Worksheet (page 189) to keep track of your progress as you put your plan into action.** Copy it, create a similar one, or go to MB-EAT.com. How you shrink up to 500 calories is up to you. It might be one big change or several small ones. Maybe you find five different ways to remove 100 calories from your daily eating, cutting 100 at each of three meals, and from two snacks. Or maybe you discover 10 ways to subtract 50. How many ways will also, of course, depend on how much your eating choices vary from day to day. But cutting back on serving sizes and on regular use of certain foods, like oils and butters, may extend across most meals.

The 500-Calorie Challenge Worksheet

Try to find at least one food at every typical meal or snack to decrease or not eat at all. Some choices are easier to implement than others. Use the easier/harder column to estimate how difficult it will be to make each change. Use what you learn to exercise your Power of Choice and make the best changes for you. Take a week (at least) to explore options, and then begin putting them into place, experimenting with even more possibilities as you go along.

Day	Meal/ Snack	Food	Amount Reduced	Easier/ Harder (1-7)	Calorie Savings	Calorie Total
	Breakfast					
	Snack					
	Lunch					
	Snack					
	Dinner					
	Snack					

Reflections on Practice 2

As you work with the 500-Calorie Challenge, try to maintain a sense of adventure and flexibility. This isn't about conforming to strict rules about how much food you can eat in any given meal or even a given day. Try to think of your food energy budget in the same way you think of your financial one: Some days you'll spend more. Other days you'll spend less. One of the drawbacks of virtually all proscribed diets is that they don't build in this flexibility. Again using money management as a useful analogy, if our discretionary money for the month is about $300, we don't use it in exactly $10 chunks per day. Some days we spend less—and then one weekend we go shopping for a new outfit or a gift. Similarly, if we decide to reduce that discretionary budget, we still don't systematically spend less every day of the month. As long as you stick to a rough calorie budget on a weekly or monthly basis, you'll do fine, but it does need to add up to your goal amount over a reasonable period of time if you want to see weight-loss results.

Maybe, you find, you can easily eat half a piece of pie when at home, but when you eat with your parents, it's easier to eat a whole piece than to deal with comments about why you're only having half. A man in one of our groups decided to take out all of the three to four regular sodas he drank most days. He then realized he really wanted at least one, so he decided to cut out more of other foods. However, by the end of the 10-week program, he was drinking only diet sodas, as he was now finding the one regular soda too sweet. Someone else substituted skim milk for half-and-half in her coffee at home, which felt virtuous but unsatisfying. She then did the calorie calculations and realized that, when spread out over 3 cups of coffee, at about 2 tablespoons per cup, she could go back to 2 percent milk, which provided some of that creamier experience. This saved her almost 80 calories over the half-and-half, a healthier and more satisfying compromise, yet added up to only 15 calories more than the skim milk. But if all that was available for coffee at a meeting was half-and-half, she used that without worrying about it.

This also isn't about "being good" until you lose the weight and then returning to your old way of eating. Rather, it's about making permanent changes that you feel you can live with indefinitely, and finding foods that are worth giving up or reducing to get to a healthier and more comfortable weight.

PRACTICE 3

Spread Out Your Food Energy

It's midafternoon and you're hungry. What should you do? Should you ignore your hunger and try to last until dinner? Or should you listen to that gnawing sensation and have a snack? And if you opt for a snack, how large of a snack is best?

This practice will help you tap into the outer wisdom needed to make these types of decisions. As reviewed earlier, depending on your metabolism and body size, you need 100+ calories per waking hour to power all your hungry cells. If your goal is 1,600 to 1,800 calories per day, and you're awake 16 to 17 hours a day, you can divide your calorie needs per day by those hours, and it comes out to about 100 calories per hour. Note that the heavier you are—whether because you are overweight, tall, or muscular—the more energy you need for your goal body weight because every cell in your body wants its allocation of food energy. But the 100 calories per hour estimation can still be helpful. If it's less than what you actually need, either increase it somewhat or allow yourself to feel a little hungry, knowing that your hunger is a sign that you are burning some excess weight.

Let's try to use this so you can make better choices about how much you eat and how often.

The Practice: Spreading Out Your Food Energy

1. **Set a rough 100-calories per hour budget for yourself.** For example, you might decide to eat a 500-calorie breakfast at 7 a.m. Because you know 500 calories will likely keep you satisfied until noon, you'll know that you probably don't need a morning snack. Or perhaps that feels like

too large a breakfast. So you might want to save out a piece of fruit for a 10 a.m. coffee break. At noon, if you opt for a 400-calorie lunch, then you can expect to start feeling peckish around 4 p.m. and may need a snack if dinner is still a few hours away.

2. **Look for instances when you feel physically hungry and it's not time for a meal.** Think about what you've already eaten and when you ate it. Also consider how many hours will go by before your next meal.

3. **Then decide on an appropriate snack.** For example, if dinner is 4 hours away, you might choose to have a 300- to 400-calorie snack in the midafternoon, and then remind yourself to try to eat a slightly larger lunch when dinner is going to be that late. And rather than feeling guilty, keep in mind that you are simply giving your body the fuel it needs to last until dinner. If you go without a snack, what will happen? You may begin dinner feeling ravenous. Your hunger overpowers your ability to eat mindfully, and you gulp down more food than you truly need to feel satisfied. Or maybe you start nibbling, beginning a chain reaction that doesn't stop until many hours later.

Reflections on Practice 3

This practice isn't about robotically eating because it's time to eat based on the 100-calorie-an-hour guideline. The point is to accept what your body is telling you and to give yourself permission to have a reasonable amount of food to get you through to your next meal, rather than beating yourself up for being drawn to more food than a single piece of fruit or a handful of carrot sticks, which won't keep you satisfied until your next meal several hours later. You still need to tune in to your hunger, and you also want to tune in to fullness and satisfaction. People in our workshops consistently tell us how helpful they find the 100-calories per hour guideline. Allow all of your wisdom tools to work together to help you decide what and how much to eat.

PRACTICE 4

Eat More/Eat Less: The Alternative to Food as Poison

Nutritional and medical science have provided a growing amount of evidence during the last 80 years regarding the health benefits of certain foods and the health risks of others. This has translated into dramatic increases in evidence-based recommendations regarding healthier diets and the development of valuable guidelines, whether expressed as official recommendations by the USDA, as nongovernmental recommendations by the American Medical Association and the Academy of Nutrition and Dietetics, or as training programs such as Jim Gordon's Food as Medicine movement. We would all do well to keep this information in mind as we choose the foods we serve ourselves, and our families.

Over the years, though, we've all been told to stay away from certain foods for all sorts of reasons. In the name of good health, we've all been told to cut out trans-fats, sugar, processed foods, red meat, and desserts. You've probably seen or even tried to follow the advice to *never* . . .

- Have soft drinks. They are liquid poison.
- Have *any* refined sugar. It too is poison.

- Consume wheat gluten. It inflames all the cells in your body.
- Eat snack chips. They're addictive and you'll never be able to stop at just one.

This advice is difficult to follow, especially if you happen to love bread, the occasional soda, or chips.

An alternative is to engage ways to add more—perhaps a lot more—healthy foods into your diet and that of your family, while retaining more appropriate amounts of less nutritious foods that you really love.

Can you have the foods you love and still be healthy? Of course you can. It all comes down to outer wisdom.

The Practice: Eat More/Eat Less

For this practice, you'll try to notice when you might be susceptible to the food-as-poison mind-set and instead learn how to make your own nutritional decisions to add to the outer wisdom you've been cultivating. To do so:

1. **Spend some time learning about nutrition.** What foods promote good health and why? You might consider using the USDA's MyPlate as a starting point (see ChooseMyPlate.gov). It was developed by a team of experts to reflect current knowledge of nutrition and health. The following are recommendations based on the MyPlate guidelines:
    - Half of your plate is composed of produce. Fruits and vegetables are loaded with vitamins, minerals, and health-promoting nutrients. And good news: frozen vegetables retain most of their nutrient values. Fruits and vegetables also offer a lot of volume for the number of calories.

- A quarter of your plate is grains, and at least half of those grains (on average, across the day) are whole grains such as oatmeal, brown rice, buckwheat, millet, bulgur wheat, barley, or foods made with whole grain flour. Whole grains contain the entire kernel—including the bran, germ, and endosperm—whereas refined grains often lack the bran and germ, which contain most of a grain's nutrition and fiber. Fiber also slows digestion and helps manage blood sugar levels, resulting in longer-lasting satiety. Overweight women who substituted whole grains for refined grains lost more fat when they followed a low-calorie diet than did women on a similar calorie diet, but without whole grains.[1]

- A quarter of your plate is protein, or about 5 to 7 ounces a day, which represents all the protein you need for good health. Plant-based protein foods—such as peas, beans, soy, and seeds—may be the most filling because they contain fiber to slow digestion. Two or more times a week, consider seafood as your source of protein, as it is higher in health-promoting omega-3 fatty acids and generally lower in calories than red meat.

- Dairy products, such as milk or yogurt can accompany meals, with an emphasis on lower-fat options. They provide calcium, vitamin D, potassium, protein, and other health-promoting nutrients. Lower-fat varieties reduce your food energy intake. But you might decide that low-fat cheese just isn't worth it, whereas a smaller portion of higher-fat, premium cheese hits the spot. Experiment!

Keep in mind that the image of a plate is not necessarily applicable for many meals, or types of foods, nor is it intended to be. For example, a nutritious sandwich with a side salad can fit the MyPlate guide, as can a bowl of chili with more beans than meat (or perhaps vegetarian), served with a salad and perhaps a whole wheat roll. Some of our workshop participants on limited budgets have also raised concerns about eating in a more healthy way, not realizing that making whole grains part of a main course can actually be inexpensive.

You are welcome to continue to explore the world of nutrition as you'd like. The vast majority of people I've worked with, however, have found room for improvement of their personal food choices based on the MyPlate guidelines alone. They find that they could easily include more vegetables and less meat, more whole grains and fewer refined foods, and so on.

2. **Take the nutritional knowledge you gained and use it to set three nutritional goals** that make sense for your health and the inner wisdom you've already cultivated. The following are some of the goals my workshop participants have come up with:
    - Trying something new from the produce department each week.
    - Targeting a certain amount, such as $20.00 (or more), to spend each week on fresh fruits and vegetables.
    - Eating one extra serving of produce every day.
    - Trying whole grain pasta.

- Eating whole grains (brown rice, quinoa, bulgur) twice a week.
- Switching from whole milk to 2 percent milk.
- Greatly reducing servings (and serving sizes) of high-sweet/high-fat desserts and snacks.

3. **Once you've incorporated three goals, add a couple more.** Keep doing this until you feel more confident that you are eating a balanced range of foods that fuel your body, promote good health, *and* satisfy your taste buds.

4. **Continue identifying sources of high-fat, high-sugar, highly processed foods, and high-salt foods** (especially packaged and canned foods) in your typical daily or weekly intake. Then consider ways to be more discerning. Engage the eat more/eat less guideline: more healthy foods, and less of others, but not the all-or-nothing, food-as-poison approach that is often touted. Where can you cut back? Reduce your serving size of desserts (without reducing your pleasure, because your taste buds let you know that only a few bites are really enough)? Use healthier oils to sauté foods? Treat yourself, perhaps, to one piece of fried chicken, not three? Buy the lower-sodium variety of foods such as tomato sauces?

5. **Keep an eye out for current health and nutritional information that is relevant to you and to your family.** Are you particularly susceptible to diabetes? To cancer? To heart disease? To rheumatoid arthritis? High blood pres-

sure? Look for new information pertinent to preventing or managing those health issues, as you create patterns of eating that are both sustainable and satisfying.

Reflections on Practice 4

Be gentle and generous with yourself. You've spent many years developing food preferences and shopping and cooking habits. They don't have to change overnight. Experiment, take some classes, and check into alternatives. Engage your family in the eat less/eat more perspective, and gradually try to move in the directions that you'd like.

Moving On

You may be surprised to find how many ways you can engage your outer wisdom in developing a more balanced relationship to food. Even if you've been on uncountable diets, you may discover new ways to relate to food and your own energy needs that are far more subtle, and certainly more fun. Rather than focusing solely on calories, food energy simply becomes one of the many aspects of choice you have. It won't always seem easy, especially at first, but you can begin to let these choices flow more, rather than being a constant source of worry or concern. You may find that even when you're eating to comfort yourself, small amounts of your favorite foods can still fit into your overall caloric budget, just as small splurge purchases may fit into your financial one.

CHAPTER TWELVE

Exercising Your Power of Choice

You've now worked your way through the fundamental building blocks of inner wisdom and outer wisdom. You can now begin to combine them to start making choices that work better for you and are flexible yet balanced overall. Let's say you're hungry and you want a snack. Will it be the corn chips or the carrot sticks? The cookies or ice cream? You're at a restaurant and want to start with an appetizer. Which calls you more—the crab cakes or the fried shrimp? Should you plan to share it or have the whole amount? Your favorite fast-food place is offering a special. Do you super-size it or decide to get what you usually do?

How do you make such decisions? The answer: You exercise your Power of Choice. The practices in this chapter will show you how. These practices start with choosing between two similar nutritious snack foods and then become more challenging, reflecting the wide variety of choices we're faced with every day. You can spread these practices out over several weeks or even longer and can repeat them over and over again as you wish, always with a sense of exploration, curiosity, and self-acceptance.

Exercising your Power of Choice is a simple two-step process that you can do quickly in your mind. You just need to stop a moment to consider:

What is calling me? What do I really want to eat? These questions are liberating for many people, mostly because, for years, they've been telling themselves what they *shouldn't* eat as well as what they *should* eat. Alternatively, they've also been mindlessly grabbing whatever food is nearest or most convenient. The practices in this chapter will help you to take a breath, step back, and consider, when you're reaching for food: Do I really want this? Do I want something else? What would I find most satisfying right now? How much might I want?

Why is it calling me? What is influencing my decision? These questions help us break out of the "I should" and "I shouldn't" thoughts that can drain all the joy out of eating: "I should order the side salad because fries are so fattening." "I should eat the rest of what's in front of me or my friend will think I don't like her cooking." "I should eat my vegetables, but I don't like broccoli." Your "why" might be simple: "It's what's calling me more." Or it might be more complex: "I'm really hungry. It looks satisfying, and I think it would keep me from feeling hungry again for several hours so I can concentrate on this important work project for the rest of the afternoon." By considering why you want to eat a particular food, you'll become aware of all of your "shoulds" and your automatic reactions: "I always eat this." "I should have it because it's the healthiest option." "It's cheaper than the other options." "Everyone else is having it." "It's there."

And yes, outer wisdom is also important. You do want to consider how many calories are in a food, and there may be times when your budget, your health, and your relationships are also important factors to consider. But you want to bring all of those considerations into balance, while considering what you really want and why. This may all seem like a huge effort in comparison to just grabbing something, but as you begin to engage these choices mindfully, without judgment, rather than obsessing over them, the effort will disappear. Making such choices can begin to seem comfortable, effortless—and just part of the joy of taking care of yourself and your need to eat throughout the day.

The practices in this chapter will help you shift away from obsessing to feeling empowered. You'll know that you are making reasonable, appropriate, and functional choices about what to eat and what not to eat—and that those choices are nobody's business but your own.

By exercising your Power of Choice, you will be able to:

- **Put your favorite foods back on the menu.** Rather than always defaulting to what you think you *should* eat, you'll gain the freedom to choose what you really *want* to eat.
- **Defuse your cravings and stop struggling with them.** You'll feel a lot more satisfied after eating something you want, often with a smaller serving. You'll be less inclined to go back for more because you already ate what you really wanted.
- **Stop fearing challenging situations such as restaurants and buffets.** The practices in this chapter will help you make wiser choices so you can enjoy a restaurant (and even a buffet) experience, yet still go home feeling satisfied while consuming far fewer calories.

Using the Practices

The first practice is simply a choice between two healthier foods that you pick yourself. Then you'll move to two more challenging snack foods, one sweet and one salty, in Practice 2. The practices then become more complex and challenging but reflect common situations: choosing foods in a supermarket, at a restaurant, and from a buffet. Try Practice 1 and 2 right away, perhaps followed fairly soon by Practice 3 (the supermarket) and Practice 4 (a restaurant meal). You may find, as many of our workshop participants do, that going to an all-you-can-eat buffet feels intimidating. By this time, however, you may be surprised at how different it feels going through a buffet line mindfully.

PRACTICE 1

Choose Between Two Healthy Foods

Start this practice when you're neither too hungry nor too full and when you might usually be eating this type of snack. Then choose two nutritious and similar foods, such as an apple and an orange, celery sticks and carrot sticks, two types of hummus on simple crackers, black olives and green olives, or two other comparable healthy foods. As in the previous eating practices, have at least four pieces of both available (note—for something like the apple or orange, these can be slices or chunks of each, about the right size for one mouthful). You might plan for what you need earlier in the day, or even the day before, choosing the foods, and the time to do it later. This will help you keep the decision of what to eat in the moment!

The Practice: Choosing Between Healthy Foods

1. **Put the foods, each on a separate plate, before you, and sit down.** Try to remain open to your choice and try not to choose yet.

2. **Take a few deeper breaths.** Do a mini-meditation to check in with your hunger and fullness levels, and then shift your awareness to the food itself.

3. **Look at each one.** Take in every facet of these two foods. Which one would you prefer to eat? Why? How do the tastes of the two foods compare?

4. **Take a slow breath.** Which food is calling you right now?

5. **Take that plate and put the other one to the side.** Reflect for a moment how you made that decision.

6. **Look at the food you've chosen**. Notice its shape, size, and color.

7. **Pick it up and bring it to your lips, and close your eyes.** How does it feel on your lips? How does it smell?

8. **Take a bite and chew it slowly.** What does it taste like? On the 10-point Taste Satisfaction Meter, how much taste, pleasure and satisfaction does it provide?

9. **Continue to eat, all the while noticing the smell, texture, and taste of each bite and also rating your enjoyment and**

satisfaction on the Taste Satisfaction Meter. Try to enjoy this as much as you possibly can. Continue to savor the food until you've either finished it or no longer wish to eat any more. Notice any surprises in this experience. Any regrets with your first choice perhaps?

10. **Become aware of your body.** Take a moment to rate your hunger and fullness again.

11. **Consider eating the second nutritious food**. Take it in with your eyes. Smell it. Notice how it's similar and different from the first food you ate. Do you really want it? If so, why? Then take a bite. If not, put it back down.

12. **If you've taken a bite, notice every nuance of its taste.** Continue to enjoy this second food mindfully, taking bite after bite, until you either lose interest in eating more or until the food is gone.

13. **Take a moment to appreciate the choices you've made and the food you've eaten.** Rest your hand on your stomach. Notice your hunger and fullness levels again. Notice your sensations of satisfaction now as well as any negativity, judgment, or surprises you might be experiencing.

Reflections on Practice 1

In this exercise, you practiced much more than your Power Of Choice. You also remained mindful of your hunger, fullness, and taste. And even though you practiced on a very simple food, you've already begun to understand and strengthen your Power of Choice.

Reflect on what you learned from the practice. How can it help you gain a sense of freedom around your eating? What aspect was easiest for you to remain aware of? What was most difficult? Hunger and fullness might not have shifted much, but that's okay. Did you have an urge to keep going because you thought, "This food is healthy. The calories don't count!"? Eating a whole bag of carrot sticks because they're free food may not add much to your calorie load, but it reinforces a pattern of eating compulsively. How did you make your decisions about what to eat and what not to eat? How was this practice different from how you usually make choices around food? Did you experience an urge to keep on eating? Was the practice difficult for you? What surprised you?

PRACTICE 2

Choosing Between a Sweet and a Salty Snack Food

This practice takes what you just learned to the next level. Rather than choosing between two healthy foods that are perhaps relatively similar in nature, you'll now exercise your Power of Choice over two less nutritious ones and perhaps foods you've often told yourself that you shouldn't eat.

Again, find a time for the practice when you might usually have a snack and when you are somewhat hungry, but not too hungry. Choose a favorite sweet food (perhaps a kind of cookie) and a favorite salty food (perhaps chips or crackers), this time giving yourself *more* of both foods than you think you'll wish to eat, rather than just the 3 to 4 pieces. In our workshops, we use Lorna Doone cookies and Fritos corn chips, partly because the colors are similar, as appearance might also influence your choice, but also because the flavors in each are relatively simple.

The Practice: How to Choose Between Sweet and Salty Foods

Put your snack foods next to each other on two separate plates. Then do the following:

1. **Sit down and do a mini-meditation.** Become mindful first of your breath, your levels of hunger and fullness, and then reflect on the foods in front of you.

2. **Decide which of the two you'd like to eat first.** What snack is calling you right now? How do you know? Push the other plate away so you can focus fully on the food you chose.

3. **Take in every facet of the food you chose.** Notice its shape and color.

4. **Pick it up and bring it to your lips, and close your eyes.** How does it feel on your lips? How does it smell?

5. **Take a small bite.** Chew slowly, noticing where you experience the food in your mouth and how much you are enjoying the experience. On your Taste Satisfaction Meter, how pleasurable is this treat?

6. **Continue to eat the food you've chosen, noticing the smell, texture, and taste of each bite and also rating your enjoyment and satisfaction.** Try to enjoy it as much as you possibly can, resisting the urge to swallow as long as there is still pleasure.

7. **Stop either when you no longer wish to take another bite or when you've finished the food in front of you.**

8. **Check in.** Again, rate your level of hunger and fullness.

9. **Consider eating the second option,** the one you chose not to eat at first. Look at it. Notice its shape and color. Smell it and feel its texture against your lips, but don't take a bite. How is it different from what you just consumed? How is it similar? Do you want it? If so, why?

10. **If you want it, then slowly take and chew one bite.** Notice the taste and how it changes as you chew. Take more bites if you wish, choosing to stop eating either once you've finished everything set before you or when you no longer enjoy the food.

11. **Take a moment to appreciate the choices you've made and the food you've eaten.**

12. **Rest your hand on your stomach.** Notice your sensations of hunger, fullness, and satisfaction now as well as any negativity or judgment you might be experiencing.

Reflections on Practice 2

How did you make your choices? Were there any surprises? Did you experience an urge to keep on eating? If so, why? How was this practice different from how you usually eat these less healthy snacks? If you want, check out the actual food energy (calories) you consumed and perhaps the ingredients if commercially processed. You might be surprised. For example, of the two foods we use in our workshops, Fritos corn chips have about only about 5 calories per chip, and three ingredients: corn, corn oil and salt. The Lorna Doone cookies have 35 calories each and a very long list of ingredients.

You will find that as you make choices more mindfully, you'll become more discerning. You may settle on a more favorite cookie or type of chip, and you'll also realize that by exercising choice, whether at the store before buying them or at a party before taking them, that you'll be able to savor what you've chosen with more true pleasure, rather than guilt.

FAQ

How do I help my children avoid inheriting the unhealthy eating behaviors that I'm trying to unlearn and leave behind?

The beauty of this way of eating is that you can share it with your entire family, even your children. You've been tuning in to your own inner child voice. You can take steps now to ensure your children grow up with a healthier sense of hunger, fullness, satisfaction, and joy. As you are choosing what to eat, make comments like, "Do I want an apple or perhaps a banana?" "Do I really want a hot pretzel now? Or would I rather wait until later when I'm hungry and likely to enjoy it more?" And while you're eating a dessert, you might note, "Oh, three bites was just perfect. I'm not really tasting it much anymore, except it's too sweet now." During a meal, you might set your fork down and push your plate away, noting, "I think I'm getting full. That's enough!" In addition to modeling balanced choices, you can nudge your children toward mindfulness with comments like, "Are you really physically hungry now? Or is it eye hunger?" and "Oh, let's save the pie for later; we'll enjoy it more then."

PRACTICE 3

Exercise Your Power of Choice at the Supermarket

Many of us shop on autopilot, grabbing the same foods we always grab. When we do stop to make careful choices, those choices are often based on our budget. We buy something because it's on sale or because we have a coupon. We may not stop to ask, "Which one of these do I really want more? Which one looks most appealing? Which one will I likely enjoy the most?"

Yet, just by asking these kinds of simple questions, we're likely to *save* money, even if we end up buying a more expensive item. How many times have you bought something because you had a coupon or because it was on sale, only to have it sit in your cabinet uneaten for months? Or you've gulped it down, barely getting any pleasure out of it? You really haven't saved anything then.

Similarly, taking time to consider what you really want can also help you eat less for all of the reasons you've already discovered: When you consume the foods you really like, you'll end your meals feeling more satisfied and less likely to reach for something else.

Of course, we shop on autopilot for a reason. The number of choices can be overwhelming. The cereal aisle alone offers scores of options. If we carefully considered what we wanted in every single aisle, we'd be there all day.

That's why, for this practice, you'll devote your mindful awareness to one type of item that you frequently buy. Maybe it's cereal. Or perhaps it's frozen dinners or apples or cheese. Choose the category and then, instead of buying the one you always do, take in all of the options and consider what looks most appealing and why.

Think of your venture as an experiment, one that is not unlike a wine tasting. When wine connoisseurs do a tasting, they fall in love with some wine and simply don't care for others. They see a tasting as a fun way to discover new wines, not only and not as a way to test their accuracy at choosing good wines. Try to cultivate a similar mind-set about your grocery store experiments.

The Practice: Exercising Your Power of Choice at the Store

1. **Set a weekly experimentation budget.** How much you devote to mindful experimentation is up to you. Maybe it's $5 or $10 or $20. Give yourself permission to spend this money each week on discovering new foods.

2. **Staying within your budget, purchase a sampling of one type of food.** So if you're experimenting with apples one week, buy a few different ones. Or if you are experimenting at the deli counter, ask if you can have a few small samplings—just a slice or two—of several different types of cheese or lunch meat.

3. **Take your sampling home, and try them to see which one you enjoy the most.** As you do so, use all the other skills you've already learned.

4. **Experiment with more foods over time.** If you started in the produce department, perhaps continue with your ex-

perimentation at the deli counter, the pasta shelves, the frozen vegetables, and beyond.

Reflections on Practice 3

As you experiment in a wider range of sections at the store, you'll be happy that you did. Sure, you might purchase a few duds on occasion, but you'll also discover many new foods, varieties, and brands. Some might be so appealing that you feel satisfied on much smaller amounts, saving yourself money and calories. For instance, workshop participants have told me that the intense taste of expensive cheese is so satisfying that they eat much less of it than the cheaper, less flavorful varieties. It's the same with dessert and snack foods. They are a lot less likely to eat the whole bag or box when they take time to discover and then choose what they love the most.

Similarly, you might also find that some foods are not as out of reach financially as you might have believed. So many people with limited incomes tell me that they can't afford to buy fresh fruits and vegetables. When I challenge them to experiment by spending $20 in the produce section, though, they often report, "I didn't realize how much I could buy with that amount. For the price of one fast-food outing for my family, I bought enough fruit for almost a whole week." And they end up healthier and happier for it.

PRACTICE 4

Choose What Foods to Eat at a Restaurant

Now you'll strengthen your Power of Choice even more by eating in a setting where you have many, many options: a restaurant. For this practice, it doesn't matter what style of restaurant. It can be fast-food, casual, or finer dining (though preferably one with larger servings).

Many people are intimidated by eating out, often because the diets they are following have scolded them to be wary of restaurant fare: Too many calories! Too much fat and salt! The portions are too big, and you won't be able to stop yourself from overeating!

But while eating out might be challenging right now, it doesn't have to be. Once you learn how to exercise your Power of Choice, you'll be able to choose a meal that you want and stop eating when you've consumed the amount that you want.

The Practice: Exercising Your Power of Choice at a Restaurant

While at the restaurant:

1. **Consider what you will order.** (*Note:* You can do this step at home if the restaurant has an online menu.) What menu items do you want and why? Is this something you truly want? Or is it merely a meal deal? If the latter, consider which you want more: To save a little money and order a meal that contains hundreds more calories than you really need (such as the fried fish special) or to pay a little more for something you truly want to eat? As you mindfully consider this choice, you just may find that this isn't a black and white, either/or situation. Is there a way to order something you really want *and* save money *and* consume a smaller portion?

   For example, one of my workshop participants often mindlessly ordered the largest burger along with supersizing the fries and a soft drink at a fast-food place. But when she ordered mindfully, she realized that what she really wanted was a smaller burger, small fries, and a glass of water. The price was a little less, she enjoyed her meal more, with no guilt or discomfort afterward, and she consumed almost a thousand fewer calories. Even then she would sometimes leave part of her burger or fries. Over the following year, she lost more than 50 pounds, partly from making these kinds of choices.

If you are ordering food at a sit-down restaurant, consider whether you want to start with an appetizer and a salad or just one or the other or neither? Are you in the mood for chicken or fish or red meat or pasta? Do you really want the bread that comes with it? And do you really want to finish what the wait staff sets before you? Or perhaps you'd still enjoy the meal if you ate only a third or half of it, saving the rest to take home.

2. **As you make these choices, use the skills you've already learned.** Consider your level of hunger. Consider how large a meal you need or want. How long since your last meal? How long until your next? Perhaps you really need only a lighter meal—and so decide to ask the waiter to recommend the best soup. You might want to add a side salad and then share a dessert.

3. **Interweave mini-meditations (eyes open is okay!) throughout the meal.** Use a moment or two of breath awareness to rebalance and check in.

4. **Once your meal comes, continue to exercise your Power of Choice.** How much do you want to eat? Do you want to consume everything presented, including your main course? Do you want to take some of it home to enjoy later?

5. **Take a few bites, but remember to slow down.** Then check in with your Power of Choice again, but informed by how much you are enjoying the food in front of you. As you eat, check into your Taste Satisfaction Meter, savoring each bite, but then reflecting: Do you want to continue eating? Do you want to stop eating that food and move on?

6. **As you continue to eat, check in regularly with hunger, fullness, and body satiety.** Do you want to save room for dessert? At what point are these experiences telling you "enough"?

7. **Continue to exercise your Power of Choice.** Do this until the last enjoyable bite.

Reflections on Practice 4

What did you take away from this practice? Consider how it can help you make more powerful choices in the future while eating out. Did you have an urge to keep eating something that you really didn't want? Why or why not? How did you make your decisions about what to order and about what to eat and what not to eat? How was this practice different from how you usually eat at a restaurant? Was the practice difficult for you? What surprised you?

PRACTICE 5

Choosing Quality Over Quantity at a Buffet

So many people fear buffets, often because they've been cautioned to stay away from such places. They've been told that the food is terrible or warned that they'll never be able to stop eating. Others have learned to manage buffets only by being "very good," heaping on the more nutritious foods and never going back for seconds—while they sadly watch their companions return again and again to the buffet line.

We're often faced with these kinds of situations, whether it's the large number of choices at a salad bar, at a community or family potluck, on a cruise, at a hotel breakfast buffet, or even at a retreat center. We're left to decide: What do I take? What do I leave? How do I choose? Do I go back for seconds?

One of the first clients I worked with using some of these approaches was older, widowed, and loved going on cruises. She was also very overweight (more than 300 pounds), and had been told by her cardiologist that going on another cruise might be too dangerous, given her heart condition—but she had already paid for her next cruise. We worked on tuning in to hunger and fullness, and on making mindful choices. She shifted her perspective from "eating all I can" at the buffets to using them as an opportunity, as she put it, to be "very, very picky." She came back gleeful. Instead of gaining weight during the cruise, as she always did, she lost a few pounds, and her blood pressure was closer to normal. A year later she had lost over 100 pounds, and she was still going on cruises.

So if you remain aware of your Power of Choice, you really can walk into a buffet or all-you-can-eat situation of any kind, choose the best of the best, enjoy every bite, and walk back out feeling victorious, energetic, and pleasantly satisfied, but not stuffed to the point of discomfort. Rather than opting for quantity, again go for quality. This is a special opportunity to eat small amounts of a number of foods and then go back for more of only the ones you really want. It allows you to experiment and find which foods you really love and which ones you don't.

This practice will show you how.

The Practice: Exercising the Power of Choice at a Buffet

Go to a buffet restaurant of your choice. It might be a casual buffet, the fancy Sunday one at a nearby hotel, or just the Chinese or Indian buffet down the street. The first time you do this, you might want to pick a buffet that you are comfortable going to by yourself, so you can practice making your choices and eating in silence to help focus your awareness—and enjoyment.

Again, be realistic about choosing a good day and time. You'll possibly be eating a somewhat larger meal than usual, so take that into account.

This practice has five core elements: check out all the offerings, sample small amounts mindfully, give yourself permission to go back for seconds, plan to leave food on your plate, and enjoy! You might want to jot these down on a note card to take with you to the buffet.

While at the buffet:

1. **Take a walk around the buffet and check out all the offerings.** Which ones are calling to you? Which ones do you think you would enjoy the most? Why do you feel this way? Notice whether you feel tempted to take more, just to get your money's worth. Notice whether this thought comes up repeatedly during the meal.

2. **Decide which foods you wish to eat while planning to go back for seconds.** Going back for seconds may seem frightening, but it's what actually gives you back power and control. Start by helping yourself to what seems to be the best of the best—the foods that are calling you the

most. You can take small amounts (perhaps three bites worth) the first time, have the plate removed (along with those foods that just weren't what you hoped for), and go back for seconds of the most delicious ones. Do a third or even fourth trip, until you've had a little taste of whatever might appeal. (And save the dessert selections for later—but you might look at them now, so you can decide how much room to save for that part of the meal.)

3. **Notice whether you find yourself avoiding foods you consider to be fattening, such as fried foods, despite yearning for them.** Also notice if you end up putting some healthier foods on your plate just because they are low in calories, even though you don't particularly want to eat them right now. If you don't really want them, leave them at the buffet. On the other hand, if you *do* want them, by all means, put a few on your plate.

4. **After making your choices, sit down and sample what you have, using all the mindfulness tools you've already developed.** Tune in to hunger, taste, and enjoyment. As you sample, consider these questions: Are there any foods that looked amazing but that failed to live up to expectation? Are there others that taste even better than you anticipated?

5. **As you eat, check gently into your hunger levels, your fullness levels, and your body satiety experience.** Don't let the challenge of the buffet lead you to forget to check in to your body's messages.

6. **Stop eating each food once you no longer wish to continue** (because it didn't taste as good as it looked) or when you've finished that small portion.

7. **Go back up for whatever was best,** for a little bit of other foods perhaps, but this time, plan to leave some food on your plate. This gives you the freedom to choose more and to stop at enough.

8. **As you eat, make careful choices about which foods not to eat more of and which ones to continue to eat.** And of course, continue to check into your hunger and taste satisfaction, and as you continue to eat, your fullness level. Again, give yourself permission to go back yet another time as you wish.

9. **Then go back to repeat this process for the dessert table**—if you want to.

Reflections on Practice 5

How did you make the choices you made? How do you feel about those choices? What could you do differently in the future to feel more satisfied in similar situations where many choices are available? How aware were you of your hunger, taste, fullness, body satisfaction, and enjoyment? This buffet experience makes almost everyone who takes our workshops very nervous ahead of time. Yet afterward, there is a sense of huge accomplishment and excitement. How can this new wisdom help you to make more powerful choices at dinner parties? Potluck events? What can you welcome back into your life? For instance, perhaps you now can join your friends on that cruise that you've been afraid of going on because of the ever-present buffet meals.

Moving On

In this chapter, I've given you increasingly difficult challenges, but don't limit yourself only to these. Continue to practice and exercise your Power of Choice as much as possible. As you do so, your awareness will increase. Try eating sometimes in silence and at other times when surrounded by friends. How do these changes in surroundings affect your choices? Continue to experiment with different foods, different surroundings, different levels of hunger, and different amounts of foods.

After each eating adventure, consider how you did. How aware were you of your hunger, taste satisfaction, tastefulness, body satiety, and enjoyment? How did you make the choices you made? How do you feel about those choices? What could you do differently in the future to derive more satisfaction in similar situations where many choices are available?

Over time, you'll find that your ability to choose becomes faster, more ingrained, and more powerful.

You may get to the point where you see a delicious food and you think, "I want that, but I don't want it right now." This realization can apply in many places: at home, at a social gathering, at a dinner party, or at a restaurant. By exercising your Power of Choice, you'll not only be able to choose the treat you want the most, you'll also be able to choose when, where, and how much of it you eat.

CHAPTER THIRTEEN

Balancing Emotional Eating

Eating for emotional reasons often gets labeled as the primary culprit for unbalanced eating. By now you know that is only partially true. But mindfully managing emotional eating can be particularly challenging.

This chapter will lead you through practices to help you better understand your own particular stress-eating patterns, how these can set off chain reactions of overeating, how comfort eating can become part of balanced eating, and when to look for other ways of coping.

How quickly you move through the practices in this chapter depends a great deal on how out of balance you feel you are with emotional eating. As discussed in Chapter 2, nearly everyone eats in response to emotions from time to time, but for some, those emotional triggers have become overwhelming. In fact, emotional eating can be a balanced, healthy way to celebrate a success or soothe the ache of a loss. It's normal to eat as a form of comfort, to calm down or to take your mind off something. Many people do it, even those who consider themselves to be slim, happy, and in balance around food. Then they'll go on to use other ways to cope.

So my wish *isn't* for you to eat only because you are physically hungry. That would both be unrealistic and unnecessary. Rather, after you read this chapter and complete the practices, it's my hope that you'll be able to eat in a more balanced way that includes sometimes using food to celebrate, comfort, or reward yourself and to handle anxiety or anger, but to realize you can do so without feeling out of control. To find that place of balance, you may need to spend several weeks or more with these practices, doing them over and over again until they feel familiar. Or you may need to do them only once because you are already pretty balanced in this respect.

In either case, the practices will teach you how to decide when it's appropriate to eat in response to emotions, when it might be better to surf your emotions as if they were waves, or when it's best to cope in noncaloric ways, perhaps by venting to a friend, picking up something to read, or going for a walk instead of eating. You may also realize that you need more assistance in dealing with the underlying emotional issues, whether or not you're able to bring your emotional eating into better balance.

You really can decide to eat out of emotional hunger and choose the foods you decide to eat mindfully. It's possible to do this without going overboard, and without feeling guilty, weak, or worthless.

That's mindful eating, and it may be very different from your current way of eating. No matter how out of balance you may feel related to emotions and eating, the practices in this chapter will help.

The Benefits of Emotional Awareness

With the help of the practices in this chapter, it's my hope that you'll be able to:

- **Learn to distinguish better emotions from real hunger.** Some emotions, like anxiety, mimic hunger so much that it can be hard to tell the difference. With mindful awareness it's easier to do so.
- **Experience more freedom to choose to eat or not to eat.** Often emotional eating follows a pattern. A negative emotion (anger, sadness, loneliness, guilt) leads us to the refrigerator, either to soothe and comfort ourselves or to avoid thinking about our problems. These practices will help you hit the pause button, so you realize you have many choices for handling such feelings and only one of them is eating.
- **Let comfort food actually bring you comfort.** When you use food to comfort yourself, actually let yourself get comfort out of it rather than getting more upset, with thoughts like "I'm a terrible person. I can't believe I went and did this again." Instead, you'll be able to eat a satisfying amount, thinking, "That was fantastic. I feel better now. I can move on and take care of this problem."
- **Learn how to surf the urge.** By observing a sense of craving mindfully and without judgment, you can ride it out until the wave drops down, rather than crashing on your head. With more experience, you'll find you can ride out larger and larger waves—or cravings!

- **Ditch the "I've Blown It" effect.** As mentioned earlier, the "I've Blown It" effect goes like this: You eat something. You feel guilty and even more uncomfortable. So you eat more, and feel even guiltier. You think, "Now I've blown it. I might as well keep on going." With the practices in this chapter, you'll learn how to interrupt this vicious circle *at any point.*
- **Increase your awareness of emotional triggers.** An urge to eat may be a window into realizing that emotional distress—anger, anxiety, depression—is actually behind it. Perhaps these triggers really do need further attention from a professional therapist, or perhaps you can, in letting go of eating as a primary way to cope, find other ways to handle these emotions. Or both.

Using the Practices

It's important to stay with Practice 1 long enough to better understand how your emotional experiences and eating are related. Then, once you feel confident with that practice, Practice 2 and Practice 3 can be done in quick succession or even concurrently. Spend enough time with the first three practices to build confidence in using other coping tools before moving onto Practice 4.

PRACTICE 1

Identify the Links: Your Eating Patterns and Emotions

In doing this practice, try to turn off the critical part of your mind that labels yourself as bad. Instead, do this practice with a sense of exploration, trying to just notice how your emotions play a role in your eating choices and patterns. The focus for this practice is just exploring patterns that may be there, rather than trying to change any of them.

The Practice: Identifying the Links Between Emotions and Your Eating Patterns

In the next week or two, make it your goal to identify 5 to 10 times when you use food to cope with an emotion.

1. **Whenever you notice yourself feeling angry, depressed, bored, anxious, or another emotion, pay attention to how you decide to cope and seek comfort.** Is your first urge to reach for food? If so, what food? And how much food?

2. **Similarly, when you find yourself eating when you are not really hungry, try to identify whether an emotional trigger led you to the kitchen, café, or vending machine.** It might be something entirely different—social pressure, taking a break, an ad on TV—but check in mindfully with your experience. What are you feeling? Are you also anxious? Angry? Depressed?

3. **As you identify these patterns, consider whether certain foods are linked with particular emotions.** For instance, you might find, as one woman I counseled did, that your late-night eating has nothing to do with hunger and everything to do with anger. And that she always wanted chocolate.

4. **As you explore these triggers, take note of when you experienced the emotional trigger, the food you were**

drawn to eat, and how the experience went. Did you feel better when you ate? Or worse? Could you consume a small amount and move on? Or did a small amount lead you to eating a larger amount? Did you go for foods you loved? Or were you consuming foods that didn't even taste all that great? Your answers will help you to build wisdom and understanding.

If you want to make notes on these patterns, you can do so, either in diary format or by creating a simple form like the one on page 226.

Reflections on Practice 1

Are there any surprises? What did you notice? Not every emotion is going to link with eating, nor is every time you eat out of balance going to be linked with an emotion. You may realize more fully, as we've discussed throughout the book, that there are indeed a range of triggers for eating and for wanting to eat. But when emotions play a role, it's always valuable to notice and identify them. You may have also noticed that only certain emotions link up to a desire to eat, and they need not be at very extreme levels. It might just be mild anxiety or mild frustration. If so, you can readily look for other coping options, ride the wave of the emotion (see the next practice), or simply accept the pleasure and comfort of the food (without it triggering off a binge), and *then* look for other ways to address the issue. Or you might begin to realize that indeed every time you have a craving for something in particular to eat (often a sweet), it is a signal that a more serious issue is still nagging at your mind and heart, and perhaps you need to seek help resolving that issue.

Understanding Your Emotional Eating

If you wish to keep track of your emotions and eating patterns, you can create a simple form similar to this one, which was filled out by one of my clients. She rated her desire to eat on a 1 to 10 scale. Or copy this one. Or you can simply tune in, and jot down notes in a journal to keep track of your patterns.

Day and Time	Situation	Feeling or Emotion	Desire to Eat (1-10) and Type of Food	Food Eaten or Other Choice
Friday, 2 p.m.	At work	Frustration	4—crunchy snack	Went to vending machine; got chips
Friday, 9 p.m.	At home—watching TV	Angry at son	8—ice cream	Had about 2 servings, then stopped
Monday, 10 a.m.	At work	Anxious about project	5—Doughnuts in break room	Looked at doughnuts, did mini-meditation, and then made to-do list

PRACTICE 2

Surf the Urge

In the first practice, you explored your eating patterns, but you were not focused on changing them. In this practice, you'll take things a step further by trying to insert a pause between the emotional trigger and that first bite.

Strong emotions and cravings can feel scary, like something that requires an immediate response. But they are nothing more than an intense inner experience, and as many of my clients have found, they are often the gateway to wisdom. If you sit with a strong emotion or a craving for a while, you can learn to hear the messages they are telling you rather than needing to immediately react to them.

The Practice: Surfing the Urge

Try this practice whenever you feel a strong emotion or a strong urge to eat, especially when you are not physically hungry.

1. **Pause.** Breathe a few times with awareness. Try to sit with the emotion. Study it. How does it feel? Where do you feel it in your body? How intense is it? Pay attention to the thoughts that travel through your mind. Listen to them, but don't react to them.

2. **Notice how strongly food calls you now that you are feeling this emotion.** If you feel strongly pulled, where in your body do you feel this sensation? How intense is it? What food do you yearn for?

3. **Do not judge any of this.** Just pay attention and observe without reacting. You are learning to pay attention to the

thoughts, the feelings, the desire—all without judgment. See if you can mindfully watch this urge until it dissipates. Note that if the feelings are very strong, it might be hard to just sit with them, so you might want to do something else that is not too distracting at the same time, such as a household chore, as long as you keep checking in with your feelings. But it's better to develop the ability to just sit with the feelings and then watch as they drop down. Just observing strengthens both your awareness and your ability to ride the feelings out without reacting, which current neuroscience is suggesting actually weakens the strength of such emotions in the future.

Reflections on Practice 2

As you get used to surfing the urge, you'll be able to use an urge to eat as a signal to tune in. You'll notice that you're about to go for the chips, and you'll consider, "What's really going on here?" That's when you might notice that you are upset about an argument you had with a coworker. In this way, the very urges that, in the past, have triggered your eating can instead let you know to be more mindful, and more in balance. The urge to eat is itself a signal to pay attention to what else is going on (for example, wanting something crunchy means anger; wanting a brownie means rebellion; wanting ice cream means sadness). Again, this connection may occur for relatively minor, day-to-day ups and downs, or it could perhaps indicate something floating under the surface that deserves to be brought out into the light and explored with the help of a professional.

PRACTICE 3

Expand Your Comfort Routine

It can be perfectly normal to turn to a small amount of food as a source of comfort, but you don't want food to serve as your *only* or primary source of comfort. After all, some problems can linger for hours or days. If food is the only way you know how to cope with the usual stress of the day, much less something like the loss of a loved one or a job, you'll be turning to food almost 24/7 and, as a result, have a very difficult time managing your weight or getting into better balance with food. So it's important to cultivate other coping strategies.

The Practice: Expanding Your Comfort Routine

1. **Make a list of alternative coping strategies to consider when you are triggered to turn to food.** Come up with several options that might give you similar comfort that you're currently searching for from food. Your list might include any of the following:
   - *Other distractions:* These might include playing a computer game, engaging in a hobby that's easy to pick up, or reading. As you create your distraction list, try to think of activities that are the functional equivalent to eating in regard to time and effort. So, let's say you usually head to the vending machine during a break at work. What else might get you away from your desk or your worry about work for a few minutes and that's easy to do? Reading a magazine story? A walk around the office or around the block?
   - *Calming activities:* If you eat to soothe anxiety or anger, make a list of alternative activities that would accomplish

the same goal. Maybe you could do the breathing meditation from Chapter 7. Or you might take a nap or call a friend just to chat.

- *Coping activities:* Rather than using food as an escape, consider facing the problem head-on. What are some things you might do to help you gain perspective or courage? Try coming up with a game plan or calling a friend to talk through the concerns.

2. **Once you have your list of activities, lean on it as needed.** Stick with it until you feel more confident in the balance between emotions and eating.

Reflections on Practice 3

As you surf your urges, you'll become more and more aware of your chain reactions and learn to lean on your comfort routine, naturally gaining a sense of freedom and mastery. You'll turn off your automatic reactions, and you'll be able to make honest, mindful decisions about your eating. Sometimes you'll surf the urge, the urge will pass, and you'll just get on with your day. Other times you'll decide that you'll have a small treat, savoring every bite. Then you'll get up and solve the problem that triggered you. Over time, you more easily handle smaller stressors and, in doing so, reinforce the new, more balanced patterns.

And you might find that certain patterns seem really hard to let go of completely. One person I worked with had been struggling for years with eating late in the evening, along with a glass or two of wine, before going to bed. This had been a typical binge time for her. She no longer binged, but now she felt she shouldn't be eating at that time at all. She'd tried to follow the evening abstinence rule: No food after 8 or 9 or even 10 p.m., but she just couldn't stay with it for more than a few days.

She realized this pattern went back to sneaking food as a teen (I could resonate with that), and it still felt a bit rebellious and self-indulgent, which she admitted she liked. So I asked her to take a week and just track how much she was eating and how much wine she was drinking, as well as some of her feeling and thoughts.

As it turned out, between about 9 and 11:30, depending on when she went to bed, she took in between 400 and 600 calories most nights. This surprised her, as she'd assumed she'd been eating much more than that.

She decided to be more creative during that time: limiting the wine to one glass, picking out intensely flavored snacks that felt really satisfying in small amounts, putting those snacks into small dishes, fully acknowledging her sense of treating herself, and enjoying the taste along with a savory dash of rebelliousness. As she described to me how much she was enjoying this, she almost laughed! She was able to get the calories down to under 400 while she embraced her pattern of enjoying this food. And she had let go of the struggle completely. Several months later, she realized that simply being present with these feelings and accepting them had shifted their power. Her desire to eat late at night had not only weakened but had gone from nightly to only a couple of times a week. And she'd lost about 5 pounds without any other effort.

You can do the same, especially if, every step along the way, you're making a conscious choice—one that is informed by your mindful awareness.

PRACTICE 4

Identify the Chain Reaction

Eating in response to emotions can be quite complex and involve extended chain reactions that you may not even realize are happening. The chain reaction looks something like this:

1. Something unpleasant happens that brings up negative emotions.
2. To feel better and to comfort yourself, you eat.
3. As you eat, you begin to feel guilty, which makes you feel even worse.
4. So you eat some more.
5. The more you eat, the worse you feel.
6. When you eventually stop eating, you feel much worse than when you started *and* you've overeaten.

Here's where you can gain some freedom: At any point in the chain, *you can break the cycle.* At any point, you can start over. There is no such thing as blowing it. It's never too late to stop eating. Even if you've eaten seven cookies, stopping at seven is better than continuing until the whole box is empty.

The Practice: Identifying the Chain Reaction

You may wish to do this practice with pen on paper, so you can see what your chain looks like. Use the Chain Reaction Cycle on page 235 as a guide for doing this.

1. **Think back to a time (the more recent the better) when you ate more than you wanted,** perhaps eating well past the point of comfort. What happened in the time that led

up to your eating? What time was it? Where were you? What was going on around you? Were you alone? Or with others? How were you feeling? What did you start eating? How were you feeling while you were eating? How were you feeling afterward? What kinds of thoughts were running through your head? Were you being critical of yourself? Were you being judgmental?

2. **Use your answers to create a Chain Reaction Cycle.** Start with what triggered you to eat, starting off your cycle. You can begin with the major links and then go back and fill in the smaller steps. Then, one link at a time, include as many sequential steps as you can, outlining what led to more and more eating. Include the thoughts that you had, how you felt, and what you did.

3. **As you fill in each link in the chain, tune in to the thoughts you were having then and consider whether they were helpful.** Were your thoughts helping you get in balance with your eating? Or were they taking you in a different direction?

4. **Try to be attuned to the distorted thoughts that you use to justify eating something** when you're not really hungry but are actually emotionally upset. For example, "I deserve this." "I'll show you." Or "I've had a bad day."

5. **Consider whether there are other ways to address those thoughts that don't involve eating.** For example, if you've had a bad day, maybe you deserve a comforting, or even decadent, treat. But is it possible that you also deserve to

relax and watch your favorite television show? Go shopping? Or pick up a book or magazine? Take a walk through the park?

6. **Look for places to break the chain.** You can be as creative and flexible as you wish. Look at the Chain Reaction Cycle and think about where this person might have interrupted her growing struggle—perhaps by finding another person to talk to at the party, indulging in only one or two brownies, or coming up with something else to do at home. You can interrupt the chain anywhere!

The Chain Reaction Cycle

When recording your own Chain Reaction Cycle, use the sample form here—filled in by one of my clients—as a guide. It's helpful to begin with a number of the key links in the chain—and then fill in smaller links in between as you think of them. Your links can include physical sensations, thoughts, emotions, and surrounding events. You can always include additional links or fewer links. Consider what you might do differently in the future to interrupt the chain reaction.

Went to a party and felt ignored by an old friend.
Felt hurt and angry.
Felt drawn to the snack table for comfort.
Started eating the brownies.
Felt better.
Kept eating.
Still felt angry!
And guilty for eating so much!
Ate more at home!
Finally talked to a different friend and felt better.

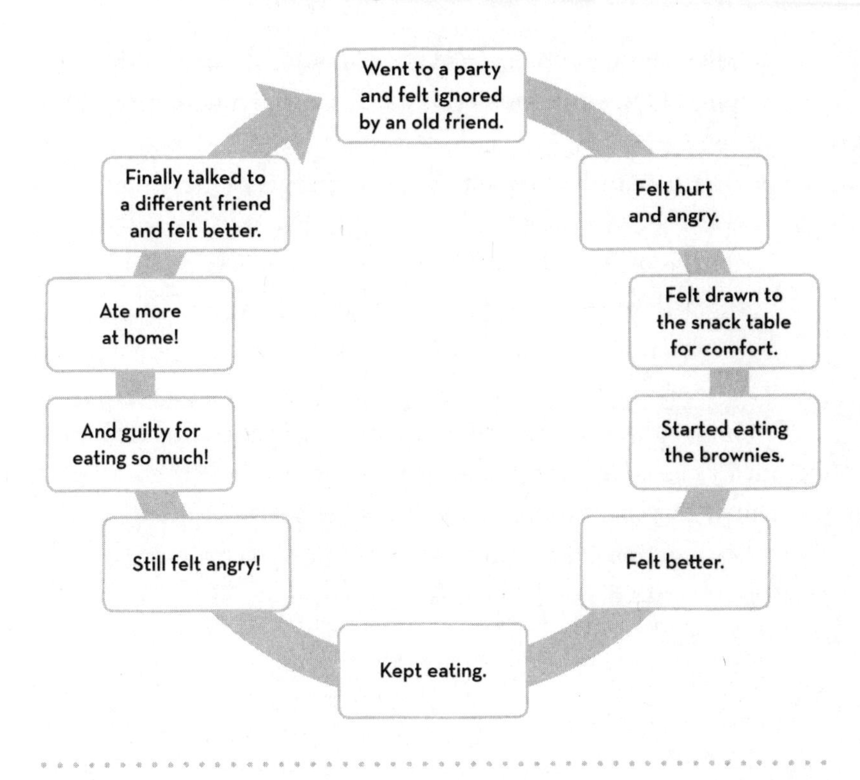

Reflections on Practice 4

Now that you've identified one chain reaction, you're ready to practice looking for others until the process comes naturally to you. In the future, when you find yourself feeling emotional or notice a strong urge to eat when you are not physically hungry, consider stopping and drafting out a new chain of links. This can help you remember when to take a mindful breath, think of alternatives, and get back into balance sooner.

Several times this week try to identify the following:

- **A stressful event as it happens:** Note the thoughts, emotions, and sensations or reactions in your body. Then check to see if those reactions create any impulse to eat. Consider alternative ways to comfort yourself. There is no single right answer.

- **Other situations that act as eating triggers:** These might include social situations, seeing tempting food, boredom, and so on. Again, identify the thoughts, emotions, and physical reactions surrounding this situational trigger. Tune in to your wise mind, and again, look at your options.

As you continue to practice, be gentle with yourself. This is not intended as an opportunity to beat yourself up. Rather, it's an opportunity for you to learn more about yourself and your thinking and about your emotional and eating patterns. Once you understand your patterns, you can firmly tell yourself, "I don't have to do this. I can stop this cycle."

FAQ

When I try to think back to a time when I overate, I start feeling the same strong emotion that led to the eating and the same strong guilt about the eating. What should I do?

Take a break and do a little breathing meditation. Remind yourself that you are learning valuable and important things about yourself and that this awareness will help you gain freedom around your eating. Practice experiencing this emotion as a wave: you can let it break over you and sweep you along or you can simply stay with it, riding it, until the wave crests and then falls. This emotional situation is clearly significant for you, and you may need help—just not food—for dealing with it. You might also choose to find a less powerful emotion to first work with to create the chain reaction practice. Or if you stay with the more intense emotion, rather than going right to the chain reaction exercise, start by just jotting down a few notes, perhaps for five minutes (you could set a timer), and return to the exercise again later, perhaps for five minutes at a time, until you can simply observe these sets of experiences without them feeling so overwhelming.

Moving On

You've now gained solid experience in creating more balanced eating and developing all the core elements of inner wisdom: tuning in to physical vs. emotional hunger, knowing when you've had enough, and knowing how to more fully enjoy your food without eating it mindlessly or contaminating that pleasure with guilt and fear. As you practice, you'll discover more ways to bring yourself into a healthier relationship with your eating and food, gaining more confidence that you can deal with the challenges in your life without the need for cartons of ice cream or bags of chips. But a small bowl or crunchy handful, enjoyed mindfully, still might be a nice part of taking care of yourself.

FAQ

I've done everything you suggested, and I still can't stop myself from late afternoon eating. What am I doing wrong?

It might be that, in addition to experiencing distressing emotion, you're also overly hungry. In the late afternoon, you might be frustrated and starving. You might also be exhausted. These triggers often intertwine with guilt, making it difficult to manage your eating at that time.

To overcome the guilt, grant yourself permission to eat in the late afternoon. After all, if you had a light lunch, you possibly *are* hungry, and it's perfectly reasonable to eat something. If you remember from Chapter 5 and Chapter 11, you need to give your body enough fuel to make it through the day. So if it's 4 p.m. and you are planning on eating dinner in three hours, a 200- to 300-calorie snack—such as a slice of bread with peanut butter, or several cookies, or some low-fat frozen yogurt with fruit, *or* ½ cup of your favorite rich ice cream—is perfectly reasonable. But that handful of carrot sticks probably won't do it.

Use all of the skills you've already learned as you consume your snack. Be mindfully aware of your changing hunger, fullness, and taste satisfaction. Then, once you finish eating, start surfing the urge and using the other practices suggested in this chapter. In this way, you can combine your inner and outer wisdoms to eat a reasonable amount of food without going overboard.

CHAPTER FOURTEEN

Deepening Your New Relationship with Eating and Yourself

You've been eating for a very long time, ever since your first year of life. By now you recognize how many of your habits and patterns have become both mindless and out of balance. And you're shifting them, by using your new mindful eating skills, in a direction that helps you let go of some of the effort and the struggle. Now your ability to eat mindfully can continue to strengthen as you find new ways to enjoy food more, while eating less. It's a lot like learning to play a musical instrument: difficult to begin with, but as you continue to play, you realize how much you're enjoying it as you also become more and more skilled.

One day you may realize that it is no longer difficult to keep the pint of your favorite ice cream in the house because you usually simply don't *want* more than a few bites at a time. Or you order steak at a restaurant, and it's *easier* to leave half of it to take home than it is to finish it. Or you go to a buffet and leave not only feeling comfortable but pleased because of the variety of dishes you had a chance to sample.

You may realize that a food that was previously a binge trigger doesn't even seem appealing. Or that the challenging situation of a family holiday has become relaxed, rather than a constant struggle between overeating and criticizing yourself.

Every time you notice such changes in your life, that's when you'll know that mindful eating is becoming part of your lifestyle. It's with you to stay.

Making permanent change is the most important aspect of this plan. So, whether this is your first attempt at slimming down or your fortieth, I want this to be the beginning of a new direction that not only lasts but deepens.

Your Relationship to Your Eating, Your Weight, and So Much More

You have been working with those many decisions you make about your eating each day: When? What? How much? Am I savoring my food like a gourmet or wolfing it down mindlessly? You are feeling successful every day as you realize more and more of these decisions are healthy and well-balanced. You might realize you've enjoyed a whole meal, while socializing, without overeating and without obsessing and are left feeling perfectly comfortable afterward. Creating a better relationship with your eating will lead to a healthier weight, so gradually the scale will follow.

In just a short time, your relationship to eating has already changed. You've learned how to tune in to taste, fullness, hunger, and pleasure. You may be moving more. Perhaps you've learned some surprising information about nutrition and food energy. You've cultivated inner and outer wisdom. And you've freed up energy for other things in your life.

Maybe you are now:

- **Maintaining a regular meditation practice.** Even 10 to 15 minutes a day helps you stay in better balance and connect with your inner wisdom.
- **Using mini-meditations.** Often our group participants, even months later, tell us that using mini-meditations regularly was the most powerful tool for tuning in to hunger, taste, fullness, and other inner experiences.
- **Eating mostly only when you feel physically hungry.** But not at the expense of turning down that exotic food you rarely have a chance to eat or refusing your sister's homemade pie at Thanksgiving. Healthy eaters are flexible eaters; you might just eat a little less at your next meal or skip a later snack.
- **Putting small amounts on your plate and giving yourself permission to go back for more if you are still hungry.** You've learned you can be flexible!
- **Savoring every bite.** Appreciate the power of your taste buds. Why keep eating something if you're not enjoying it? It's easy to use mindfulness to cultivate your inner gourmet, to avoid food that you realize you don't even like very much, and to stop eating when your taste satisfaction has dropped, along with your hunger. Keep looking for foods that are worth eating, at least on occasion, and those that just really aren't worth the calories.
- **Leaving food on your plate as satisfaction sets in.** Let yourself celebrate this important ability to just leave it. And

realize that you may enjoy those leftovers more the following day, when you're hungry again.

- **Being mindful of the thoughts and emotions that trigger mindless overeating.** Awareness, without negative self-judgment, leads to wisdom and freedom. You can learn a lot from simply watching how your mind sets up those old patterns, and doing so with curiosity, rather than fear and regret.
- **Interrupting a binge or slip up at any point.** It's never too late to break the chain reaction, once you realize what's going on. You've never blown it.
- **Tuning in to the calories/food energy in whatever you choose.** Let go of the anxiety, fear, and avoidance and engage this over and over as simply very useful information.
- **Experimenting with healthier food choices.** Read articles on healthier eating—not as if they've been written by the food police but because there might be some wisdom there. Go to vegetarian cooking workshops, buy a new cookbook, try out lower-fat versions of favorite foods. Do this with an attitude of curiosity and experimentation, and not with the mind-set that if you don't meet some rigid expectation—by immediately becoming a vegetarian or vegan, always avoiding butter and oils, or completely giving up sugar—that you've somehow lost a battle.
- **Realizing there are many ways to eat mindfully.** But don't make the mistake of thinking that you will mindfully savor every bite of every single meal for the rest of your life. Mindless eating happens for everyone, especially on those days when you have only 5 minutes to gulp down lunch. Remember, a mindful lunch may be mindfully *choosing* what you have to eat in a rush; the *mindless* lunch would be gulping down twice as much as you really needed.

- **Experimenting with mindful movement.** What happens when you take the stairs instead of the elevator, park farther from where you are going, walk for 10 minutes or more a day, or enroll in an aerobic exercise program? Burning those extra calories may be part of it, but really what's important is using your body for what it's designed to do: movement. That will help you do it more and more.
- **Using mindfulness to pause for just a moment, to observe, relax, refocus your wandering mind, and engage your inner wisdom.** You'll begin to rein in the wandering mind, whenever you're worried, distracted, or daydreaming. Sometimes this state is pleasant and helpful, and you just let yourself drift there. But wandering mind also contributes to that sense of being preoccupied by your eating and weight, perhaps more often than is needed, or is helpful.

Using the Practices

No new ones for this chapter. Instead, we're returning to where you began, by checking in to your original Keep It Off Checklist and your Circle of Being. No pressure. Just check in and see where you are now.

PRACTICE 1

Revisiting Your Keep It Off Checklist

Take out and review your original Keep It Off Checklist to see how you're doing now compared with when you started this program. Each item reflects possible small steps, and you may be surprised to find just how many you've already taken. You've learned a lot as you've read through this book, and you've probably put a fair amount into practice. Where did you start? Where are you now? I think you'll find that you've been making significant progress.

You might want to copy your original Keep It Off Checklist and/or complete it again using a different color ink. Date it and put it aside again for a few months. And then plan to revisit it again.

Reflections on Practice 1

Continue to work on congratulating yourself for making small changes. There may be many opportunities to do so each day. Take a moment right now to acknowledge how far you've come. Allow yourself to be excited and pleased. Then, when you are ready, move forward a little more. For example, if you can tune in to your hunger or fullness fairly easily when you're eating by yourself, what about when you're at work? Or out at dinner with friends? Or at a party?

All the while be aware of what is and is not working for you. Not every practice in this book will have been right for you. Some will fit into your life more easily than others. It's just as important to be mindful of what doesn't work for you as it is to be open-minded about what might work. And perhaps in a few months, you'll realize you've just found an occasion to try out one of the techniques. Continue to experiment.

PRACTICE 2

Revisiting Your Circle of Being

Take out and review your Circle of Being chart from the beginning of the program. What was the percentage that represented your level of preoccupation or concern about your eating, your weight, your body? Take a moment to reflect: What number or percentage now represents that level? Has it decreased? Where would you like it to be? Consider the list you created of all the other important areas of your life: work, family, hobbies, and so on. Now as your struggle with eating has decreased, have you been able to free up energy for these other areas? How has your Circle of Being shifted?

Reflections on Practice 2

Continue to notice when the struggle with food and eating shows up again. What's behind it? When does it happen?

When I did the Circle of Being exercise with Jennifer, she initially told me that she spent 75 percent of her time worrying and obsessing over her eating, weight, and appearance. When I pressed her, asking her to consider the time she spent at work as a successful small business owner and as a wife and mother, she decreased the number to 60 percent. Over the course of working together, the number began to drop, all the way down to 35 percent, but she felt that percent was still too high. It still didn't seem balanced, even though that included grocery shopping, meal preparation for her family, eating, and clothes shopping, which now felt much more positive. However, she still wanted to think about food and her body a lot less, getting it down to just about 20 percent of her time.

I asked her, "What do you obsess about the most?"

She told me that she wanted to lose another 15 pounds by summer and that wish was very prominent in her mind. She wasn't sure she could stop obsessing about her body size if she didn't lose those 15 pounds. I was concerned because she'd also shared with me that she'd once been at a weight that I knew was on the low side for her body build and height. And that she'd gotten there by really over-restricting her eating.

I asked, "When are you worried most about those 15 pounds? Are you concerned that people notice it during a typical week, when you're at a meeting with clients, or in the office?"

"Well, no, mostly when I want to wear a bathing suit," she said.

"Do you think about it every single time you wear a bathing suit?"

"No," she reflected. "Only when I want to swim at the country club."

"Do you think about it every single time you swim at the country club?" I pressed.

"Well, no," she said. "Come to think of it, it only bothers me when Sue is also at the country club."

Sue, it turned out, was a woman she went to high school with, someone she felt envious of.

"Wow, this is really stupid," she said of her obsession to lose 15 pounds. "I see Sue only two or three times a summer, at the most."

It was after that conversation that Jennifer was able to lower her percentage from 35 percent to just 20 percent, which constituted the 3 hours or so a day she spent on meal preparation, eating, and shopping; choosing clothes, makeup, and hairstyling; and a little bit of worrying.

She was amazed. She realized she had let go of a level of worry and concern that had been with her for years.

Coping with Plateaus

Perhaps you've made quite a few changes, lost some weight, but have now plateaued. And yet your long-term weight goals are indeed realistic. How much weight you can ultimately lose will depend on many factors: your age, metabolism, starting weight, genetics, and how mindful you are of your hunger, fullness, satisfaction, and level of physical activity. However, at some point, with a given level of eating and activity, your weight loss will slow down and your weight will plateau. Rather than getting frustrated, this is a time to celebrate!

You've accomplished a real change—in eating and perhaps in increasing activity. It's not necessarily a bad idea to let your weight—and your eating—be at a balanced place for a while, as you gain confidence in the new patterns you've created. So encourage yourself.

Remind yourself that these new habits are a lot like growing plants. Watch them, keep nurturing them, and look for signs of vulnerability. Mindless out-of-balance eating can creep back in many ways. Give yourself at least several months or even more to live your life at this new weight level and to accept the gift you've given to yourself for reaching there before moving on.

Then at some point, when you are confident that you are ready for another challenge, it's time to make an important decision: Do you want to cut an additional 200 or 300 calories from your daily eating or perhaps add even more exercise? Or maybe you want to hold steady to your new habits, even if that means you won't lose more weight for now. Regardless, it is likely that your body is healthier and that you are experiencing far less struggle than before. Let that sense of self-acceptance and pride in your accomplishments grow stronger.

This is about exercising your Power of Choice. For some people, the answer is indeed eating fewer calories. They can still slice out another 200, 300, or 500 daily calories and feel satisfied during, after, and between meals. For others the answer is more exercise. They know they can bump up their daily walking or add 15 minutes to their gym time and keep it bumped up for life or, at least, for the foreseeable future. Just knowing that it's your choice to make—and not society's choice or your thin office mate's choice or your physician's choice or your spouse's choice—can help you find balance and acceptance.

You'll follow the same process as you maintain your weight. Balanced Eaters don't step on the scale and see the same weight every day of the year. Sometimes they gain a few pounds, especially during the holidays. That's normal. What separates healthy maintainers from yo-yo dieters is this: Healthy maintainers don't tell themselves, "Well, I've blown it. I might as well give up." Instead they do the opposite. They use small gains as motivation to practice healthy eating habits more consistently, and their weight comes back off.

So if you notice few extra pounds—outside of your usual fluctuations—see it as an opportunity to grow even more mindful. Ask yourself, "Was it because I'm now going out to lunch one or two more times a week, perhaps with a new friend who always orders dessert? Or is it that new bakery that opened down the block? Or have my trips to the gym gone from three times a week to twice a week? Or is it winter, so I'm not walking as much?"

You might remember that your previous reaction to this weight gain would have been to panic, and then buy the magazine at the check-out line promising to show you how to "lose 7 pounds in 7 days." Instead, here's an opportunity to stop and reflect. What needs to change to get into better balance? Yes, it can be frustrating, but we do this type of checking in for other areas of our life all the time. Have we overspent our budget by a little too much this month? Lost touch with a friend or family member? Missed a couple of deadlines at work? We step back, think about what moved us away from our intentions, consider how to make adjustments, and get back to what keeps us in better balance with our overall values and sense of well-being. This is how we can relate to our choices, patterns, and decisions about food and eating too.

Practice the Art of Forward Thinking

Your mastery of mindful eating will grow over time. Eventually, you'll get to the point where mindfulness becomes your default mode. It will be what you do most of the time before, during, and after eating. And it will feel easy to do, enjoyable, and not need any effort.

No matter whether you've already formed these habits or whether your mindfulness skills are still just growing, it's a good idea to look ahead and think about situations that might challenge you to eat mindfully.

For instance, for many people visiting their parents may be the challenge. I've had adults well into their 50s tell me, "I'm fine until I go home for the holidays!"

Indeed they are going back to the place where their mindless eating habits were developed. This is where they perhaps learned how to overeat for comfort and to mechanically clean their plates. Just thinking about eating with their parents or siblings can bring up feelings of anxiety.

For others, birthday parties may still feel like challenges. For others, vacations or the holidays or a stressful week at work is most challenging.

One strategy is to anticipate challenging situations and then plan ahead for how you will practice mindfulness during them. Even if these situations are anxiety producing, you can navigate them mindfully, using them to practice and sharpen your skills rather than abandon them.

So make a continual practice of looking ahead. What will be the most challenging eating situations for you during the next week, month, and year?

Then consider how will you exercise your Power of Choice in those situations. Maybe it's fine, for instance, to clean your plate when you visit your parents because, after all, you won't see them again for six months. Or perhaps you decide that you will be assertive and explain to your parents that you aren't hungry and don't wish to clean your plate. Or become more creative about gracefully refusing. Try saying, "That was so delicious, Mom, I'll have one more bite, but I'm really getting full!" "Can I take some home?" "You know, I'd love to make this for my husband/the kids/to bring to a potluck next week. Can I get the recipe?"

Similarly, you might decide to cultivate your inner gourmet at a birthday party by taking that piece of cake, thoroughly enjoying a few bites of it—then discreetly putting it aside, while complimenting the hostess. Or you might just have the larger piece, add on the ice cream, eat while you're enjoying the company and then mindfully cut back later in the day, because you're simply not very hungry.

At Thanksgiving you might even give yourself permission to eat to the point of discomfort, knowing that there's no such thing as blowing it and that you do so only once or twice a year. I've found that healthy thin eaters often admit that they overeat on special occasions like this! As you decide how you will navigate each upcoming challenge, ask yourself, "What will I regret *more*? Will I regret *not* having this splurge/treat/special time? Or will I regret feeling uncomfortably full for a few hours?" The answers to those questions are not the same for everyone, and they are not the same for every situation. When you make a conscious choice ahead of time, you're more likely to navigate a situation with confidence.

Make It Your Own

Part of exercising your Power of Choice lies in creating your own eating guidelines. When you try to blindly force yourself to follow the rules of any eating plan, eventually your inner child rises up and protests, "Don't tell me how to eat!"

Successful eaters are flexible. Rather than following unbendable rules, they create guidelines that fit their preferences and their lives, and alter those guidelines with their changing circumstances. They find the middle way, the wisdom that allows them to enjoy eating and nourish their bodies, minds, and souls.

For example, when I first started counseling Pam for help with her struggles with eating and her weight, she told me that she never allowed any cookies in her home. If they were there, she said, she'd end up eating the whole box. Because she didn't feel any cookie could possibly be "safe for me," she'd made a strict rule: no cookies.

Several weeks later, Pam realized she could be more flexible. Now equipped with more mindfulness skills, she felt it would be okay if she kept a box of cookies (a type she liked but didn't love) in the house, but away in a cupboard where she wouldn't see them.

Sometime later, Pam felt more confident in her mindful eating skills. She had lost some weight and was managing food temptations much better. She knew that, if she left the cookies out, she might have one or two. But she wouldn't eat the whole box. However, this still applied only to those types of cookies that she deemed safe. She still was careful that especially tempting cookies didn't come into the house.

A year later, Pam had lost about 30 pounds and wasn't binging at all. In regard to cookies, Pam's only guideline became this one: to eat them mindfully. As long as she does that, all cookies are safe with her. And those large, special bakery cookies that show up on occasion last twice as long, as she slowly savors half and puts the rest aside for later.

You will eventually get to this point, too. You might not be there today and you might not get there next week or next month, but you will get there. Eventually, as you practice mindfulness, your relationship with food will change. Rather than being a relationship with anxiety, it will be a relationship with joy. The struggle will be over, and in its place you'll find something you've always wanted: culinary delight and culinary freedom.

ACKNOWLEDGMENTS

As I've tried to express throughout this volume, there are so many mentors, colleagues, and students over the years to whom I am grateful for their contributions to my thinking, my clinical experience, and my research.

My work with individuals who are struggling with their eating and weight has informed this book all along the way. Naturally, I cannot identify by name the many, many patients who have brought me wisdom as they worked to free themselves from their struggles, but I owe them so much. My clinical mentors, of course, deserve full acknowledgment. Dr. Ferdinand Jones, at the Brown University Counseling Service, provided me an opportunity to develop and share a mindful eating group approach there. I also became involved in the Anorexia Nervosa Aid Society in Providence, Rhode Island, sharing some of this work with women who were still struggling after many years. In Boston, I had a part-time postgraduate position at McLean Hospital in the behavioral eating disorders program, under the direction of Philip Levendusky, who supported me in working with women with severe bulimia nervosa. All of these experiences laid the foundation for the clinical work I've done over the last 30 years with my clients, both men and women, who've struggled with eating disorders, particularly bulimia and binge eating disorder.

As bears repeating, the development of this approach to mindful eating had its inspiration through many years of working with notable research mentors and colleagues. Without the brilliance of those I studied with at Yale, particularly Gary Schwartz and Judith Rodin, I would have had neither the ideas nor the inspiration to move ahead as I did. Deserving particular appreciation is Peter Suedfeld, who spent only one year at Yale as a visiting professor from the University of British Columbia but whose work had inspired Gary to install a sensory deprivation chamber at Yale. One of my earliest clients, with whom I used mindful eating training, also benefited from that experience, which allowed her to deepen her inner awareness regarding both hunger and eating. Peter also supported me both personally and intellectually in more ways than I can share, encouraging creativity, broad thinking, and high-level writing. Most recently, my colleagues and friends at the Center for Mindful Eating have provided continued support and inspiration, as partners in creating TCME, in exploring many of the issues in bringing these perspectives to both the professional and general community, and in sharing their own thinking creatively and genuinely, both in print and in person. From the beginning, it's been inspiring to work with Megrette Fletcher, Char Wilkens, Jan Chozen Bays, Donald Altman, and Ron Thebarge. The group has continued to expand beyond those who can readily be listed here, but also includes Marsha Hudnall, Caroline Baerten, Lilia Grau, and Cheryl Wasserman.

Without the opportunity to learn and then deepen my own meditation practice and knowledge, this book would also not have happened. As I've noted, I first began with Transcendental Meditation in 1971, but sadly I have no idea who led me in that first experience at a center in downtown Philadelphia. After that I continued to gain experience both through the teachings of Donald Swearer at Swarthmore College and through the Himalayan Institute meditation center in Madison, Wisconsin, where I first met Swami Ajaya, a psychologist with deep training in the Hindu traditions. Their teachings provided a much broader introduction to the richness of the Hindu meditative traditions, but Swami Ajaya was the first to encourage me to link the theory that I was learning in psychology to the classic practices of meditation, resulting in my first publication in this area. I also met Dan Brown there, a psychologist who was working on his own research that linked both meditation and the theory of hypnosis with self-awareness within the Buddhist traditions of Vipassana, and who was to become my colleague and mentor at Cambridge Hospital, Harvard Medical School about 5 years later.

But this was all leading up to the explosion of interest in meditation practice in the United States, including efforts to secularize the experience of meditation in a way to make it accessible to all, regardless of their cultural or religious backgrounds. In the Boston area this was being led by Herbert Benson, whose research, beautifully articulated in his classic book *The Relaxation Response*, I drew on for my master's thesis research. And then by Jon Kabat-Zinn at the University of Massachusetts Medical Center (UMMC) in Worcester, whose book *Full Catastrophe Living* introduced to the world the power mindfulness meditation practice has to help people deal with a wide range of issues, from stress to chronic pain, anxiety, and cancer. Without Jon's work, and that of his colleagues, Saki Santerelli and Elana Rosenbaum, I might not have had the confidence to create the MB-EAT program. He has remained a close colleague and friend since I left UMMC almost 25 years ago.

This book is also deeply grounded in science. Psychology appealed to me from my first exposure due to the potential for blending human service with scientific rigor. The faculty who led me along that path included Kenneth Gergen, who taught my first introduction to psychology class and helped me conduct collaborative cross-cultural research in Japan and elsewhere in Asia; and Jeanne Marecek, who hired me as a research assistant during my final year as an undergraduate. Both have become dear friends. Becoming even more familiar with the rigors—and limitations—of the scientific method was central to my studies at the University of Wisconsin, under the guidance of such masters as Peter Lang, Dick McFall, and Howard Leventhal. And then finally appreciating the opportunity for re-immersing this rigor for methodology into the vibrant intellectual air of Yale discourse. Finally, Judith Ockene at UMMC, without whom I could never have developed the skills and perspectives necessary to conducting large-scale clinical intervention research, began as a mentor and has continued as a colleague and friend for many years.

The book, of course, would also not exist without the years of research collaboration and support I've had from so many. Shortly after I began teaching at Indiana State University (ISU), Brendan Hallett came to me, asking whether I'd mentor him for a doctoral dissertation on meditation. I responded "of course"—if we focused the project on the work I'd been developing on mindful eating. I can still remember his reluctance—"I'm a guy! I don't know anything about this!" We decided to focus the program on women with binge eating disorder, partly because of its similarities to other addictive behaviors with which he had more clinical experience. Brendan proved to be a wonderful partner in this process, helping edit the treatment manual I'd developed earlier at University of Massachusetts Medical Center, modifying it to help engage participants with a wide range of backgrounds. This research then provided the foundation for applying for our first grant from the National Institutes of Health (NIH), through the National Center for Complementary and Alternative Medicine. And that grant would not have been possible without meeting two wonderful individuals from the Duke Diet and Fitness Center, Lucy Brown and Stephanie Noll, who agreed to partner with me. Then, as the grant was funded, Ruth Wolever, author of *The Mindful Diet*, replaced Stephanie, who was moving on to another position. Ruth has been a friend and a partner in developing this work ever since. The project itself moved to Duke Integrative Medicine, and she and her team, particularly Sasha Loring, Jennifer Davis, Jennifer Best Webb, and Jessica Wakefield, contributed substantially to many aspects of the program through additional NIH funding, particularly to development of the outer wisdom components.

My research team at ISU also made it possible, of course, to do this work, as did all the community members who participated in the MB-EAT programs over the years. When I first proposed meditation as a primary focus of my teaching and research, shortly after moving to ISU in 1991, I expected some resistance. But from my fellow researchers to my chair, Virginia O'Leary, to the dean at the time, Joe Weixlmann, I received nothing but support, as has been the case from subsequent chairs, Doug Herrmann and Virgil Sheets. The research team involved in our NIH-funded trials included the staff of our Psychology Clinic, notably Jan Wright and Valinda Woods, who were forever patient and supportive, and Toni Bolinger and Kim Julian, staff in the psychology department; colleagues including June Spock, Michele Boyer, and Dr. Randy Stevens; caring and dedicated graduate students who served as group leaders and research assistants—particularly Michael Ann Glotfelter, Julie Buchanan, Brandy Dean, Joanna Ho, Anita Farrell, Janice Leigh, and Tamara Johnson; and project managers Bryland Sutton and Kelly Renteria, who rescued many challenging moments. And, of course, much appreciation to the statisticians who helped with our grants: both Virgil Sheets, wearing his other hat, and Kevin Bolinskey, whose work on assisting with complex data sets, the logistical and ethical issues of clinical trials with multiple sites, and the requirements of complex statistical analyses has been core to understanding our findings.

Since then, the projects that have been developed elsewhere, expanding or adapting MB-EAT to many other populations, have all contributed to the wisdom and value of this approach. Michael Baime and Amishi Jha led a project designed to look more deeply at neuromechanisms, also linking with the Duke University group. At Ohio State University, Carla Miller created a team to bring MB-EAT to individuals with type 2 diabetes with exceptional efficiency and clarity. At the University of California at San Francisco, the team headed by Rick Hecht and Elissa Epel has been extraordinary in their wisdom, diligence, and collegiality. Other key members of that team with whom I've worked particularly closely are Patty Moran, Jennifer Daubenmier, and Michael Acree along with many others over the last 5 years. Other projects coming out of UCSF have included inspired dialogue with Cassie Vieten, Kimberley Coleman-Phox, and Jeannette Ickovics. Finally, I want to acknowledge the dedication, energy, and patience of Andrea Lieberstein. Andrea began as one of our research group leaders and has served over the last six years as my co-leader in bringing the MB-EAT program to hundreds of individuals through professional and public workshops in the United States and in Europe. In particular, I'm thankful for Caroline Baerten and her mindful eating program in Belgium as well as many other people from the staffs of the Omega Institute, Kripalu Center for Yoga and Health, and the Esalen Institute in the United States who've provided valuable input, insight, support, and assistance.

Finally, without Alisa Bowman, this book would not exist. Not only has she been a wise and careful editor of my writing as we've gone along but she has contributed her writing skills to translating professional jargon into the self-guided practices in this volume and skillfully putting onto paper my recollections and reflections regarding both the science and clinical work. Even more important, her vision created the opportunity to move the book forward in the first place. She came across an article I'd written on mindful eating and through her agent, Michael Harriot, contacted me suggesting that we consider collaborating on a book, which has grown into this volume. Mike had worked with her on a number of previous books, including one on the *New York Times* bestseller list. And I have to express my appreciation to Mike who martialed us through the proposal stage, searching for publishers and continued to support us both in moving this to completion. At Penguin, I'm lucky to have been working with Marian Lizzi, who had previously worked with Alisa, and who has provided excellent feedback and considerable patience through all the creative steps involved.

NOTES

1. An Introduction to Mindful Eating

1 J. Kristeller, "Mindfulness, Wisdom and Eating: Applying a Multi-Domain Model of Meditation Effects," *Journal of Constructivism in the Human Sciences* 8, no. 2 (2003): 107–118.

2 B. Cuthbert, J. Kristeller, R. Simons, et al., "Strategies of Arousal Control: Biofeedback, Meditation, and Motivation," *Journal of Experimental Psychology: General* 110, no. 4 (1981): 518–546.

3 R. J. Davidson, D. J. Goleman, and G. E. Schwartz, "Attentional and Affective Concomitants of Meditation: A Cross Sectional Study," *Journal of Abnormal Psychology* 85, no. 2 (1976): 235–238. G. E. Schwartz, "Biofeedback, Self-Regulation, and the Patterning of Physiological Processes," *American Scientist* 63 (1975): 314–324. G. E. Schwartz, "The Brain as a Health Care System: A Psychobiological Framework for Biofeedback and Health Psychology," in *Health Psychology*, ed. G. Stone, N. Adler, and F. Cohen (San Francisco: Jossey-Bass, 1979): 541–571.

4 J. Rodin, "Current Status of the Internal-External Hypothesis for Obesity: What Went Wrong?" *American Psychologist* 36, no. 4 (1981): 361–372. J. Rodin, "Stimulus-Bound Behavior and Biological Self-Regulation: Feeding, Obesity, and External Control," in *Consciousness and Self-Regulation*, ed. G. E. Schwartz and D. Shapiro (New York: Plenum, 1978), 215–239.

5 L. M. Bartoshuk, "Taste, Smell and Pleasure," in *The Hedonics of Taste*, ed. R. C. Bolles (Hillsdale, NJ: Lawrence Erlbaum, 1991), 15–28.

6 S. Orbach, *Fat Is a Feminist Issue* (New York: Bps Pub, 1997).

7 J. Kabat-Zinn, *Full Catastrophe Living* (New York: Random House, 2008). J. Kabat-Zinn, A. Massion, J. Kristeller, et al., "Effectiveness of a Meditation-Based Stress Reduction Intervention in the Treatment of Anxiety Disorders," *American Journal of Psychiatry* 149, no. 7 (1992): 936–943.

8 J. L. Kristeller and C. B. Hallett, "An Exploratory Study of a Meditation-Based

Intervention for Binge Eating Disorder," *Journal of Health Psychology* 4, no. 3 (May 1999): 357–363.

9 J. L. Kristeller, R. Q. Wolever, and V. Sheets, "Mindfulness-Based Eating Awareness Training (MB-EAT) for Binge Eating Disorder: A Randomized Clinical Trial," *Mindfulness* 3, no. 4 (2012): doi 10.1007/s12671-012-0179-1.

10 J. Kristeller and R. Wolever, "Mindfulness-Based Eating Awareness Training: Treatment of Overeating and Obesity," in *Mindfulness-Based Treatment Approaches*, 2nd ed., ed. R. A. Baer (San Diego: Elsevier, 2014): 119–139.

11 C. K. Miller, J. L. Kristeller, A. Headings, et al., "Comparative Effectiveness of a Mindful Eating Intervention to a Diabetes Self-Management Intervention among Adults with Type 2 Diabetes: A Pilot Study," *Journal of the Academy of Nutrition and Dietetics* 112, no. 11 (2012): 1835–1842. J. Daubenmier, J. Kristeller, F. M. Hecht, et al., "Mindfulness Intervention for Stress Eating to Reduce Cortisol and Abdominal Fat among Overweight and Obese Women: An Exploratory Randomized Controlled Study," *Journal of Obesity* 2011 (2011): doi 10.1155/2011/651936.

2. Cultivating the Habit of Mindful Eating

1 A. Sood and D. T. Jones, "On Mind Wandering, Attention, Brain Networks, and Meditation," *Explore* 9, no. 3 (2013): 136–141.

2 J. Brewer, A. Worhunsky, P. D. Gray, et al., "Meditation Experience Is Associated with Differences in Default Mode Network Activity and Connectivity," *Proceedings of the National Academy of Sciences U S A* 108, no 50 (2011): 20254–20259. Y. Y. Tang, Q. Lu, X. Geng, et al., "Short-Term Meditation Induces White Matter Changes in the Anterior Cingulate," *Proceedings of the National Academy of Sciences U S A* 107, no. 35 (2010): 15649–15652.

3 R. Davidson and S. Begley, *The Emotional Life of Your Brain* (New York: Hudson Street Press, 2012). Daniel Goleman, *The Meditative Mind: The Varieties of Meditative Experience* (New York: Tarcher, 1996). Daniel Goleman, *Emotional Intelligence: Why It Can Matter More than IQ* (New York: Bantam, 2012). J. Carmody, G. Reed, J. Kristeller, and P. Merriam, "Mindfulness, Spirituality, and Health-Related Symptoms," *Journal of Psychosomatic Research* 64, no. 4 (2008): 393–403.

4 B. Wansink, "Package Size, Portion Size, Serving Size . . . Market Size: The Unconventional Case for Half-Size Servings," *Marketing Science* 31, no. 1 (2012): 54–57.

5 E. Tolle, *A New Earth: Awakening to Your Life's Purpose* (New York: Dutton, 2005): 75.

6 C. Davis and J. C. Carter, "Compulsive Overeating as an Addiction Disorder: A Review of Theory and Evidence," *Appetite* 53, no. 1 (2009): 1–8.

3. Connecting with True Hunger

1 B. Wansink and J. Sobal, "Mindless Eating: The 200 Daily Decisions We Overlook," *Environment & Behavior* 39, no. 1 (2007): 106–123.

2 M. Garaulet and P. Gomez-Abellan, "Timing of Food Intake and Obesity: A Novel Association," *Physiology & Behavior* 134 (2014): 44–50.

3 E. Berne, *Games People Play* (New York: Ballantine, 1996).

4 G. Alan Marlatt, "Buddhist Philosophy and the Treatment of Addictive Behavior," *Cognitive and Behavioral Practice* 9, no. 1 (2002): 44–50.

5 K. E. Heron, S. B. Scott, M. J. Sliwinski, and J. M. Smyth, "Eating Behaviors and Negative Affect in College Women's Everyday Lives," *International Journal of Eating Disorders* 47, no 8 (2014): 853–859.

6 J. Wardle, Y. Chida, E. L. Gibson, et al., "Stress and Adiposity: A Meta-Analysis of Longitudinal Studies," *Obesity* 19, no. 4 (2011): 771–778. S. Murray, A. Tulloch, M. S. Gold, and N. M. Avena, "Hormonal and Neural Mechanisms of Food Reward, Eating Behavior and Obesity," *Nature Reviews Endocrinology* 10 (2014): 540–552.

7 C. P. Herman and J. Polivy, "Distress and Eating: Why Do Dieters Overeat?" *International Journal of Eating Disorders* 26, no. 2 (1999): 152–164.

8 J. Daubenmier, J. Kristeller, F. M. Hecht, et al., "Mindfulness Intervention for Stress Eating to Reduce Cortisol and Abdominal Fat among Overweight and Obese Women: An Exploratory Randomized Controlled Study," *Journal of Obesity* 2011 (2011): doi 10.1155/2011/651936.

9 K. Blum, P. K. Thanos, and M. S. Gold, "Dopamine and Glucose, Obesity, and Reward Deficiency Syndrome," *Frontiers in Psychology* 5, no. 919 (2014): doi 10.3389/fpsyg.2014.00919.

10 J. L. Kristeller and J. Rodin, "Identifying Eating Patterns in Male and Female Undergraduates Using Cluster Analysis," *Addictive Behaviors* 14, no. 6 (1989): 631–642.

11 C. Carver and J. Conner-Smith, "Personality and Coping," *Annual Review of Psychology* 61 (2010): 679–704.

4. Full of Food, Empty of Satisfaction

1 J. E. Blundell and F. Bellisle, *Satiation, Satiety, and the Control of Food Intake* (Cambridge, UK: Elsevier/Woodhead, 2013).

2 A. Geliebter and S. A. Hashim, "Gastric Capacity in Normal, Obese, and Bulimic women," *Physiology and Behavior* 74, nos. 4–5 (2001): 743–746.

3 R. M. Puhl and M. B. Schwartz, "If You Are Good You Can Have a Cookie: How Memories of Childhood Food Rules Link to Adult Eating Behaviors," *Eating Behaviors* 4, no. 3 (2003): 283–293. B. Wansink and C. R. Payne, "Consequences of Belonging to the 'Clean Plate Club,' " *Archives of Adolescent & Pediatric Medicine* 162, no. 10 (2008): 994–995.

4 F. J. Bornet, A. Jardy-Gennetier, N. Jacquet, et al., "Glycaemic Response to Foods: Impact on Satiety and Long-Term Weight Regulation," *Appetite* 49, no.3 (2007): 535–553.

5 B. Wansink, "Environmental Factors That Increase the Food Intake and Consumption Volume of Unknowing Consumers," *Annual Review of Nutrition* 24 (2004): 455–479.

6 P. Rozin, K. Kabnick, E. Pete, et al., "The Ecology of Eating: Part of the French Paradox Results from Lower Food Intake in French Than Americans, Because of Smaller Portion Sizes," *Psychological Science* 14 (2003): 450–454.

7 M. Guiliano, *French Women Don't Get Fat* (New York: Vintage, 2004).

8 B. J. Rolls, E. A. Rowe, E. T. Rolls, et al., "Variety in a Meal Enhances Food Intake in Man," *Physiology & Behavior* 26, no. 2 (1981): 215–221.

9 E. Siniver, Y. Mealem, and G. Yaniv, "Overeating in All-You-Can-Eat Buffet: Paying before Versus Paying After," *Applied Economics* 45, no. 35 (2013): 4940–4948.

10 G. A. Marlatt, "Buddhist Philosophy and the Treatment of Addictive Behavior," *Cognitive and Behavioral Practice* 9, 1 (2002): 44–50.

11 C. P. Herman, J. Polivy, and V. Esses, "The Illusion of Counter-Regulation," *Appetite* 9, no. 3 (December 1987): 161–169. J. Polivy and C. P. Herman, "Dieting and Bingeing: A Causal Analysis," *American Psychologist* 40, no. 2 (February 1985): 193–201.

5. Cultivating Outer Wisdom

1 M. Nestle and M. Nesheim, *Why Calories Count* (Oakland, CA: University of California Press, 2012).

2 S. Agarwal, "Cardiovascular Benefits of Exercise," *International Journal of General Medicine* 5 (2012): 541–545.

3 S. C. Moore, A. V. Patel, C. E. Matthews, et al., "Leisure Time Physical Activity of Moderate to Vigorous Intensity and Mortality: A Large Pooled Cohort Analysis," *PLoS Medicine* 9, no. 11 (November 6, 2012).

4 A. Crum, J. Alia, and E. Langer, "Mind-set Matters: Exercise and the Placebo Effect," *Psychological Science* 18, no. 2 (2007): 165–171.

5 C. Werle, B. Wansink, and V. Payne, "Is It Fun or Exercise? The Framing of Physical Activity Biases Subsequent Snacking," *Marketing Letters* (2014): doi 10.1007/s11002-014-9301-6.

6. Tools for Getting Started

1 J. Kristeller, R. Q. Wolever, and V. Sheets, "Mindfulness-Based Eating Awareness Training (MB-EAT) for Binge Eating: A Randomized Clinical Trial," *Mindfulness* 5, no. 3 (2014): 282–297.

2 "Keep It Off" stands for "Kristeller Eating and Exercise Patterns of Food and Fitness."

8. Feeling True Hunger

1 G. M. Timmerman and A. Brown, "The Effect of a Mindful Restaurant Eating Intervention on Weight Management in Women," *Journal of Nutrition Education and Behavior* 44, no. 1 (2012): 22–28.

9. Cultivating Your Inner Gourmet

1 D. Zinczenko and M. Goulding, *Eat This, Not That* (New York: Rodale, 2007).

2 D. Zinczenko and M. Goulding, *Eat This, Not That! Restaurant Survival Guide* (New York: Rodale, 2012).

11. Calories: Turning Off the Panic Button

1 M. Kristensen, S. Toubro, M. G. Jensen, et al., "Whole Grain Compared with Refined Wheat Decreases the Percentage of Body Fat Following a 12-Week, Energy-Restricted Dietary Intervention in Postmenopausal Women," *Journal of Nutrition* 142, no. 4 (2012): 710–716.

INDEX

ABOUT THE AUTHORS

Jean Kristeller, PhD, is professor emeritus of psychology at Indiana State University, one of the founders and past president of the Center for Mindful Eating, and the creator of the NIH-funded Mindfulness-Based Eating Awareness Training (MB-EAT).

Kristeller has published more than 50 research articles in peer-reviewed journals, with her work gaining widespread media interest. *Self, Redbook*, NPR's "The Salt," the *Boston Globe*, the *Baltimore Sun*, and many other outlets interview her regularly and cover her research.

She presents workshops several times a year at the Omega Institute, Kripalu Center for Yoga & Health, the Esalen Institute, and in Europe.

Kristeller's interest in meditation-based treatments for eating disorders and obesity began more than 30 years ago while she was studying for her doctorate at Yale University. She went on to cofound the Behavioral Medicine program at Cambridge Hospital, Harvard University Medical School, and then continued with her clinical and research work at the University of Massachusetts Medical School. Her research on MB-EAT has been funded with multiple NIH-funded grants at Indiana State University, and jointly with Duke University, Ohio State University, and the University of California, San Francisco.

Alisa Bowman is a professional writer and ghostwriter who has penned more than 30 titles, including seven *New York Times* bestsellers. She has written for many national outlets, including *Reader's Digest*, *Spirituality & Health*, *Prevention*, *Parents*, and *Family Circle.* She teaches and practices meditation in Bethlehem, Pennsylvania, and has been a student in Jon Kabat-Zinn's Mindfulness-Based Stress Reduction (MBSR) program as well as Kristeller's MB-EAT workshop.